33 NURSES

Insight, Inspiration, and Stories from the Field

Words of Praise for *33 Nurses*

"This timely book is a precious contribution, calling your attention to the inner life work and world of nurses and nursing. In behind-the-scenes stories, we hear the call to human caring service and the call for self-caring as one act. Nurses share their personal and professional vulnerabilities as acts of courage and commitment; as acts of passion and moral values, seeking new solutions to sustain human dignity and human caring.

Each story, each moment, is a testimony to professional nurses and their heart of wisdom, compassion, love, and service, transcending panic and pandemics alike, a gift of helping us all to find solace while everything else is spinning turmoil all around."

—Jean Watson, PhD, RN, AHN-BC, FAAN, LL (AAN)
Founder Watson Caring Science Institute
Distinguished Professor of Nursing
Inducted as a Living Legend by the American Academy of Nursing
Recipient of the American Journal of Nursing's "Book of the Year" award

33 NURSES

Insight, Inspiration, and Stories from the Field

TERRY MALUK, MSPH, RYT

33 Nurses: Insight, Inspiration, and Stories from the Field

ISBN: 978-1-7327729-8-4 (eBook) / 978-1-7327729-9-1 (paperback)

Printed in USA by Terry Maluk

The publisher has strived to be as accurate and complete as possible in the creation of this book. In compliance with the Health Insurance Portability and Accountability Act (HIPAA) requirements to ensure patient privacy, there are no identifying details about any patients discussed.

This book is not intended for use as a source of health, medical, or financial advice. All readers are advised to seek services of competent professionals in health, medical, and financial fields.

Readers are cautioned to rely on their own judgment about their individual circumstances and to act accordingly.

Cover and interior design by Laurie L. Young

Cover and interior graphics © Shutterstock
Cover photos clockwise from upper left: Katie Temple, Laura Macans, Craig Metcalf, Susan Gillispie, Laurel Gibbs, Megan Patterson, LeEtte Gilbert, Jennifer.

For bulk book orders, contact
Terry Maluk
Terry@FromStressedToCalm.com

FromStressedToCalm.com

Contents

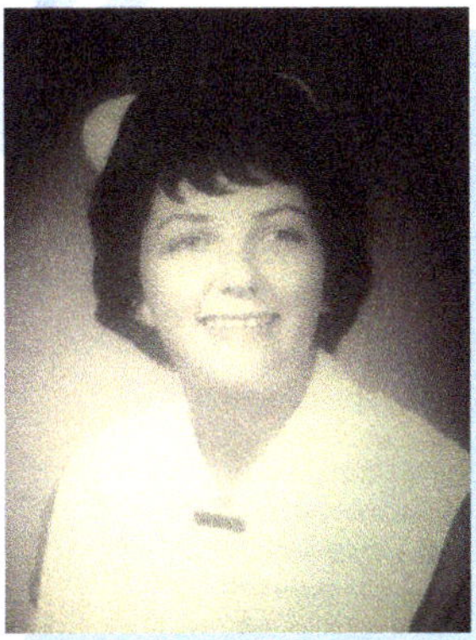

Dedication

In loving memory of my sister-in-law Jan Perkins. Your dedicated nursing career touched many lives, and your kindness and gentle smile will always be remembered.

To the thirty-three nurses from twenty-six states who shared precious time and inspiring stories for this book: Andria, Ann, Christine, Craig, Debera, Denice, Donna, Dottie, Gretchen, Jennifer, Jerri, Jessica, Karen, Kathi, Katie, Kim, Lara, Laurel, Linda Kathleen, Maggie, Mary Ann, Michelle, Morgan, Nancy, Pamela, Pauline, Peggy, Sandy, "Sandy," Sara, Susan, Tom, and Vicki. I've enjoyed working with you and getting to know you better during the course of this project. Thank you so much for everything you do.

To all nurses who step up with dedication and compassion to comfort and care for others, especially during these challenging times. Thank you from the bottom of my heart for your service.

Introduction

My introduction to the world of nurses came at an early age when my much-older brother dated and then married a nurse. My sister-in-law, Jan, was kind, caring, and always stopped to offer her full attention when we spoke, even though I was just a young child. In those years, nurses wore crisp, white uniforms, white shoes and stockings, and had white hats mysteriously secured to their heads. I loved seeing her in her uniform. Even after a long day, a smile graced Jan's face. Her daughter Jennifer followed in her footsteps, becoming a nurse and caring for others with the same dedication and compassion as her sweet mother.

The passing on of the nursing profession is a common theme among the nurses featured in this book. Whether observing a family member on the job or watching healthcare professionals care for a loved one in a medical facility, the backstories are similar. The nurses stood out with their caring touch and comforting human contact in a sea of tubing and unfamiliar, harsh surroundings. Seeing nurses doing what they do best leaves a huge impression, and those looking for a calling in life are often drawn to the medical career path of nursing.

Thankfully, there are and have been many extraordinary nurses in my life. I've learned so much about the profession and those called to serve by observing and listening to them. Nurses are a unique group of people who live to help others and to teach others how to take care of themselves.

Yet nurses are often the most resistant to practicing self-care. They choose to take care of others over taking time to care for themselves. Nurses may skip breaks, abandon entire meals, and even forfeit time to go to the restroom during their shifts so they can take care of patients. While nurses understand that proper self-care is beneficial, not only to themselves but to those around them, they often have trouble setting aside the time for even a few quiet breaths to help them regroup.

With that in mind, I set out to create a book filled with inspirational stories and advice from nurses, for nurses. The timing of the book release was initially set to coincide with the 200th anniversary of the birth of Florence Nightingale in May 2020, while also celebrating the World Health Organization's Year of the Nurse and the Midwife. Invitations went out and interviews were being conducted when the COVID-19 pandemic struck. Needless to say, interviews moved to the back burner while nurses were called to the front lines of service, risking their own lives to save others.

During the story-collection process for this book and after the pandemic struck, my dearest friend Emmi, a retired nurse, brought my attention to an article in the New England Journal of Medicine written by Dr. Heather Kovich[1] from the Northern Navajo Medical Center, in Shiprock, New Mexico. It is an eloquent, engaging piece written from the center of the COVID storm in a vulnerable place. "... the virus penetrated towns that utility companies have never managed to reach."

Given the grim, new reality, I updated the interview format from live videoconference interviews to written responses using an online form so that nurses could respond when they had time. Thirty-three nurses from twenty-six states took the time to share their stories.

Many said the process of answering the questions was therapeutic, helping them remember why they had become a nurse, provided time to review their career, and allowed them to offer their unique words of wisdom for other nurses.

The world of nursing includes many acronyms, from credentials to unit names, as you'll see throughout the stories. Where they are not defined within the story, you'll find the acronyms defined in the Glossary near the end of the book.

The thirty-three stories are primarily ordered alphabetically by state, then by first name when there are multiple nurses' stories from one state. Several nurses chose to be identified by only their first names, one chose a fictitious first name, and one chose not to share her state.

The questions were the same for each nurse with one exception: after the pandemic began, one additional question was included to ask about the impact of the pandemic on their work. For that reason, some stories do not include responses to that question.

Here are the final nine questions that were answered by each nurse who participated in this book:

1. *What made you decide to become a nurse? Was there someone or an event that influenced you?*
2. *Tell me about your nursing career, such as where you have practiced, what types of facilities you've served in, and how long you have served as a nurse.*
3. *What has been the most challenging aspect of your career in general?*
4. *Do you find the nursing profession stressful? How do you cope with the stress?*
5. *How has the COVID-19 pandemic affected your work? (Added a few months after starting to collect stories.)*

6. *Have there been times you didn't practice self-care when you knew you needed to?*
7. *What words or ideas would you offer to help nurses in their career that you wish you'd known?*
8. *What has been the most rewarding aspect of your nursing career?*
9. *Is there anything else you'd like to share with nurses that could make their lives better?*

One day, after collecting a great story from a nurse in New York, I made a quick trip to the grocery store. Holding three items in my hands, I found a short checkout line. As I waited in line, the woman in front of me moved her stuff from the front of the conveyor belt back a little bit and said to me, "You only have three things. Come up here." I noticed she was wearing scrubs, and I asked, "Are you a nurse?"

She answered with gentle confidence, "Yes, I am!" I realized she'd probably just finished a twelve-hour shift and had no time to spare, yet here she was doing me a favor that would delay her arrival home even further. I was humbled. "Thank you so much." She replied with a smile filled with warmth.

I told her that I'd been talking with nurses all over the country and writing a book about them, and I handed her my card so she could download some free stress-relief tools. We talked briefly about how nurses take care of everyone else first and, unfortunately, often put themselves last. I hoped she'd take the time to practice self-care.

After our brief exchange, she turned to the petite woman behind us and lifted two huge juice bottles out of her cart for her, and said, "These sure look heavy!" See a need, fill a need. Nurses are like that.

My friend and nursing coach Maggie Brown told me a story of needing to get out for a walk after an incredibly challenging week. There had recently been over twenty inches of snowfall where she lived. Undaunted, as Maggie always is, she set out and started walking through the fresh, deep snow. Her walk became more challenging than expected, turning into more of a trudge than a refreshing walk. She eventually reached a point where someone else had already left footsteps in the snow. Sharing the path someone else created made her journey easier. It wasn't that her foot was exactly the same size or shape as the footprints she followed, but she was thankful for the greater ease they provided on her walk.

We hope that by sharing paths and stories, the nurses featured in this book will make life easier and less lonely for other nurses on their own paths.

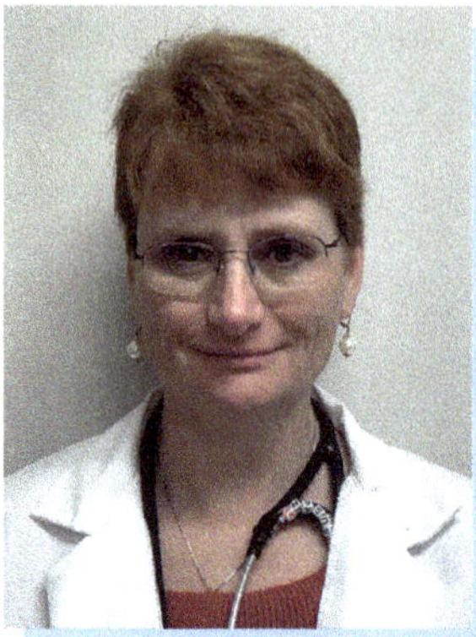

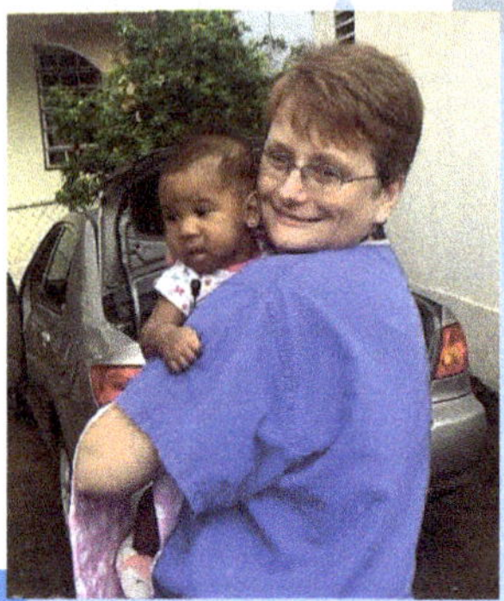

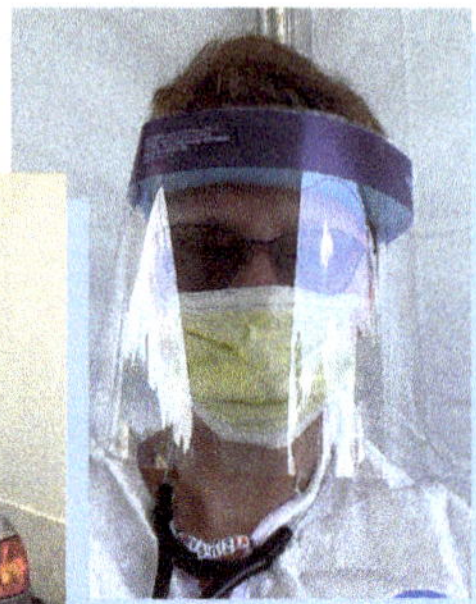

Susan M. Gillispie, MSN, FNP-C
Alabama

What made you decide to become a nurse? Was there someone or an event that influenced you?

About fifteen years ago, my husband was almost killed in a rollover accident. I was a stay at home mom with four children. I was so scared of being the sole income provider that I quickly registered for classes. I had planned on getting my degree in biology because I love biology! I thought that I would teach high school biology.

The economy took a nosedive and no one was hiring teachers. I applied to a condensed nursing program, and I got in. From a very young age, I had wanted to work in the medical field, but with my upbringing in foster care, I didn't have the self-confidence to go for my dream. With the fate of my family firmly in my hands, self-confidence no longer played a role in my decision. I had to support my family! I took to nursing like a duck to water.

Tell me about your nursing career, such as where you have practiced, what types of facilities you've served in, and how long you have served as a nurse.

I have been a nurse since 2012 and a family nurse practitioner since 2015. I had a background of being an army medic, so I had some prior medical experience. As a nurse, I worked in both home health and in the hospital on a medical/surgical floor, and as an NP, I have worked in both family practice and urgent care.

What has been the most challenging aspect of your career in general?

Being older when I joined the workforce was very challenging. I find that traditional western medicine, in which one doesn't treat the core problem and only treats the disease with medication, is very frustrating.

Do you find the nursing profession stressful? How do you cope with the stress?

Nursing can be crazy stressful! I am a person that enjoys a hot bubble bath and a juicy romance novel at the end of the day. This routine helps me wash the stress of the day away. Working with people who are sick and only getting sicker without treating the core cause is stressful for me. We live in a society where we don't want to "fix" the problem; we only want to medicate it.

How has the COVID-19 pandemic affected your work?

I have found that during COVID-19, I don't enjoy working for a large corporation. I want to spend more than fifteen minutes with a patient. I want to take the time to understand where my patient is coming from, how their illness/disease is affecting them and their family, and then together, come up with a way to improve their lives, not just prescribe yet another medication.

This pandemic has been an eye-opening experience and has led me to move forward with opening my functional health clinic[2] in January 2021. Without the stress and chaos of COVID-19, I am not sure that I would have ever made this move.

Have there been times you didn't practice self-care when you knew you needed to?

There have been many times when I was just too tired, and all I wanted to do was get home and crawl into bed. A quick shower and into bed. So, I'd grab food at a drive-through because cooking would take too long, and I had to be back in the clinic in less than ten hours. The work schedule can be daunting, and sometimes extremely difficult, especially when working the night shift. I remember one time I was so tired that I wet my bed. I just couldn't wake up!

What words or ideas would you offer to help nurses in their career that you wish you'd known?

Take a deep breath! Nursing is one of the most rewarding careers and one of the most challenging. There are so many ways to practice nursing, and not every job will be the right job. Take the time to learn about all the different aspects of nursing, try some, try them all! It is the best career, but only if you make it so.

What has been the most rewarding aspect of your nursing career?

Making a difference! Many times you don't feel that you make a difference in someone's life, then there will be that one patient. You will look back throughout your life and realize that you, only you, did something to impact that patient's life. It is amazing, and it doesn't happen that often that you can remember, but your patient will!

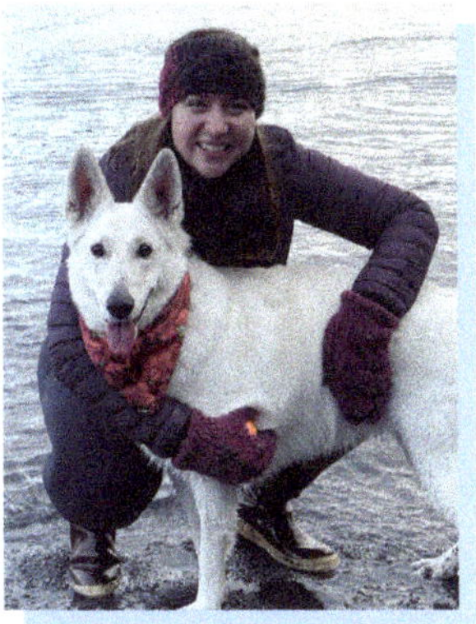

Lara Macans, BSN, RN, CPHON

Alaska

What made you decide to become a nurse? Was there someone or an event that influenced you?

I was always the injury-prone child in my family and spent my high school years rupturing my spleen, breaking my jaw and vertebrae, and generally spending more time in the hospital than a regular kid should. The adults in my life constantly told me that I should go into the healthcare field as I had so much "experience" in it already.

I was unsure of my choice to be a nurse for my whole first year of college, but that all changed the moment I got to walk into the hospital and spend my first clinical with a patient. Nurses are the heartbeat of healthcare, and I am so glad to be in a field where I'm able to care for the pediatric population in Alaska.

Tell me about your nursing career, such as where you have practiced, what types of facilities you've served in, and how long you have served as a nurse.

I work at Providence Alaska Medical Center on the inpatient pediatric unit as a pediatric oncology nurse. I have worked there for six years.

What has been the most challenging aspect of your career in general?

Working in pediatric oncology, we get to know many of our patients over several years of treatment. We know their families, the names of their stuffed animals, and what they want to be when they grow up. The most challenging part of my career has been when those kids don't get to grow up. I have had to learn how to cope with that death in a healthy way that allows me to be a good nurse still and to continue living a vibrant life outside of the hospital.

Do you find the nursing profession stressful? How do you cope with the stress?

Nursing definitely can be stressful! Having actual lives in your hands is challenging and can feel like playing a high stakes game all day for twelve-plus hours.

My best advice is never to forget to reach out for help when you need it. Reach out to your fellow nurses for an extra hand, work closely with your physicians, coordinate care with that physical therapist, ask the pharmacist about that med. Healthcare is a team sport, and you should never feel like you have the entire weight of patient care on your shoulders.

Have there been times you didn't practice self-care when you knew you needed to?

Absolutely. I believe self-care is a skill you need to practice! For the first few years of my nursing career, I often took work home with me and would find it hard to sleep after a bad day at work. While taking work home with me does occasionally still happen, I've gotten better at taking care of myself. Schedule that massage, book your next get-away, and go for a walk outside after a hard shift.

What words or ideas would you offer to help nurses in their career that you wish you'd known?

Never say never! I said I would never be a nurse until I was in nursing school. I said I could never be a pediatric nurse, and here I am, a pediatric oncology nurse, and I LOVE it. Always be open to where your nursing career takes you, even if it's not the traditional path.

What has been the most rewarding aspect of your nursing career?

That's an easy one. My pediatric oncology patients are, hands down, the best part of my career. Watching them kick cancer's ass, watching them grow up, playing "we are the champions" as their last chemo infusion finishes.

I also love teaching new Peds oncology nurses in our APHON course. It's a blessing to train the next generation of Peds oncology nurses and see them grow to love these kids just as much as I do.

Is there anything else you'd like to share with nurses that could make their lives better?

You make a difference!

Pauline, APRN, PMHNP-BC

Arkansas

What made you decide to become a nurse? Was there someone or an event that influenced you?

Becoming a nurse seemed like a natural thing for me because my mom was a nurse. I watched her go to work daily and was greatly inspired by the difference she made in our community as a nurse, and I made a vow to myself to be like her. She also encouraged me to follow in her steps, so I had her support from the beginning.

Tell me about your nursing career, such as where you have practiced, what types of facilities you've served in, and how long you have served as a nurse.

I graduated from nursing school in May 2011. I started on an orthopedic floor, moved on to neurology, cardiology, then psychiatry.

I've been a nurse for nine years now.

What has been the most challenging aspect of your career in general?

Balancing family life and career, but I would not trade it for anything.

I find my work fulfilling and my family supports me. I just have to make sure I plan ahead, so I don't miss out on my children's activities and milestones.

Do you find the nursing profession stressful? How do you cope with the stress?

Nursing can be stressful at times, but not always. It feels good knowing that you play an important role in positively impacting a patient's life for the better.

To de-stress and balance my life, I exercise regularly and meditate. Self-care as a nurse is critical because you can't pour from an empty cup.

How has the COVID-19 pandemic affected your work?

I worked on a surgical floor during the pandemic, so initially, there were many work cancellations, which caused financial strain. I took the time off to spend time with my family as my kids adjusted to virtual courses.

We have since resumed work, and taking precautions at work has been of the utmost importance because I want to protect myself and my family while still providing care to those affected by this devastating disease.

Have there been times you didn't practice self-care when you knew you needed to?

Most definitely, and this resulted in burnout. I found myself getting irritable very quickly and not being the nicest person in the room.

I have since learned to take breaks and time off from work because my body needs rest and rejuvenation.

What words or ideas would you offer to help nurses in their career that you wish you'd known?

Be kind to yourself.

You will make mistakes. It's okay. Learn from your mistakes and do better.

What has been the most rewarding aspect of your nursing career?

Having patients come back when they are well to say thank you. It gets me every time. Just knowing I made a difference for the better makes me content.

Is there anything else you'd like to share with nurses that could make their lives better?

Always be kind, and don't take things so personally. You never know what someone is going through.

Christine, RN
California

What made you decide to become a nurse? Was there someone or an event that influenced you?

In my career as an environmental scientist, I started to feel too distanced from the results of my actions. I was looking for something where I could see the impact of my work directly.

I'd been practicing yoga for about a decade and was also drawn to being of direct service to my community. I had volunteered in our local emergency department, where I met several great nurses who encouraged me, and I went through several of my own hospitalizations with wonderful nurses.

As my parents age, I also wanted to know how to best care for them, if the need arises. Nurses are so tough and competent, and I wanted to be like them!

Tell me about your nursing career, such as where you have practiced, what types of facilities you've served in, and how long you have served as a nurse.

I work at a small community hospital in Humboldt County, northern

California. I became a nurse at age fifty-three after a career in environmental science consulting. I've worked as an RN now for two years, at the same place, on the medical/surgical unit.

What has been the most challenging aspect of your career in general?

Getting everything done fast-fast-fast because there's always more to do than there is time to do it. Seeing that other nurses seem to, somehow, get everything done and have plenty of time on their hands and can stand around and chat. Dealing with the challenges of COVID-19 and the evolving hospital policies around it. Caring for patients who are repeatedly self-harming with drugs, alcohol, poor eating, and lack of exercise and self-care. Staying positive when other nurses are critical or harsh.

Do you find the nursing profession stressful? How do you cope with the stress?

Yes, very much so. You have to get so much done so quickly, but also safely and with compassion. I try to have a sense of humor, which I can share with patients to some extent, and laugh with other nurses about the crazy things that patients do or say, about things the hospital administration is doing, or about the deplorable state of health care in general in this country. If we didn't laugh about it, I would despair.

At home, I do a lot of gardening, food storage, and cooking. I do yoga and take walks and hikes with friends. I get massages. I listen to audiobooks and connect with my book club, which is now meeting online.

How has the COVID-19 pandemic affected your work?

Luckily COVID-19 numbers in my county, and at my hospital, are relatively low (so far). At first, I was pretty upset about the apparent lack of real-time and stockpiled reserves of PPE, and we were just getting by the best we could. Then our hospital was able to catch up to a degree, which has taken some of the stress off.

When we have a patient for whom we are waiting on a COVID-19 test result, we treat them as if they have it, so that involves a lot of extra steps and PPE, which for nursing staff means a lot of extra time, and for the patient, it means a lot less contact, as they are in isolation. And the hospital-wide ban on all visitors means that all the patients are feeling more isolated, and the nurses need to do more phone communication with family members who are worried about their loved ones.

As the pandemic expanded, people with nonemergency needs stopped coming to the hospital, so our patient count went way down, which has put a financial strain on the hospital (it's privately owned), resulting in furloughing of staff. I haven't been furloughed, but it's especially hard to get your job done well when the support staff of nursing aides is cut way back.

Have there been times you didn't practice self-care when you knew you needed to?

Especially this year, with COVID-19 and the social upheaval, I know I spend too much time online looking at news and social media, taking away time that I could be spending outdoors or exercising indoors with an online group, or reading for pleasure.

I still work part-time at my old job, as well as my full-time nursing job, so I'm still very busy even while sheltering in place. I've put off needed preventative medical and dental appointments because I get my care out of the county, in an urban area, and I don't want to make the long trip into a highly COVID-affected area.

What words or ideas would you offer to help nurses in their career that you wish you'd known?

To new nurses, I would say that the first year is rough because you don't really know what you're doing. That is just a given, so don't feel bad about it. Every week you will get better and better at the job. Make mental and physical notes about mistakes you made, or see others making, so you can remember what to do better next time. Rely on the aides for help and help them out when you can.

To experienced nurses and managers, I would say that how you treat new nurses makes a critical impression on them, positive or negative. Nearly all the nurses at my hospital have been gracious and helpful, and some have been especially encouraging and helped me understand the practice of medicine and the operations of the institution where I work.

My preceptor was exceedingly kind and knowledgeable, and we shared many laughs, especially when I did something particularly clueless and realized it. The camaraderie of experienced nurses makes the stress of learning a new profession tolerable.

On the other hand, the established nurses who are curt or bossy or unkind or intolerant really ruin a person's day and make a new nurse wonder why they are busting their butts so hard just to be treated rudely.

What has been the most rewarding aspect of your nursing career?

It's fun to learn a whole new field, to learn technical information, skills, and approaches to caring for people. Most patients are very appreciative and kind and make you feel good for helping them effectively while they are in a vulnerable state. It's rewarding when you know that during your shift, you advocated for a patient, or effectively taught them information they can use to advocate for themselves or corrected a mistake or misunderstanding in their care. I like sharing information with new RNs, aides, and students, and encouraging them in their career development. It is gratifying when you really connect with a patient, come to like them, and make them feel safe.

Is there anything else you'd like to share with nurses that could make their lives better?

I would encourage nurses to practice self-care regarding the most obvious factors I see in the nursing population: to quit smoking and to keep off too much weight. I hate to think about the long-term consequences of these health problems on my fellow nurses, which I realize are probably coping mechanisms for a busy and stressful life. But I want them to live long and happy lives!

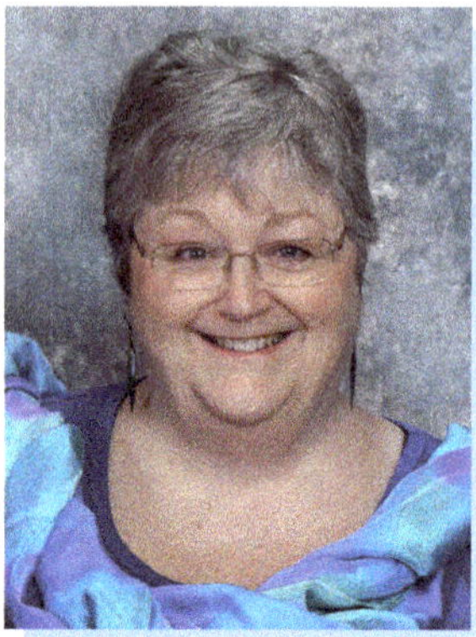

Dottie Shields, The Psychic Tapper, EFT Practitioner, RN, CMT

California

What made you decide to become a nurse? Was there someone or an event that influenced you?

When I first went to nursing school, the choice was teacher, secretary or administrative assistant, or a nurse. I chose to become a nurse because I thought I wouldn't have to write papers in nursing school! But I made the right choice, because as it turned out, I was a nurse for forty years. I am a healer.

Tell me about your nursing career, such as where you have practiced, what types of facilities you've served in, and how long you have served as a nurse.

I became a nurse in 1971 and started going to psychic classes in 1978 and joined a psychic program in 1979. That's when I found out I had healing capabilities with my hands. I learned that my vivid imagination about people was actually my intuition, and after all these years, I still trust my intuition.

I learned hypnosis in a basic program. Then in the early 2000s, I studied acupressure at the Acupressure Institute in Berkeley (which no longer exists) and completed their basic 150-hour program and then completed two 200-hour specialization trainings. One of my specializations is in pain management and one is in stress management. In California, acupressurists are certified as Certified Massage Therapists (CMT), as the practice is hands-on.

In 2014, I started learning EFT (Emotional Freedom Techniques) with Rob Nelson in Santa Rosa. He taught both EFT and Matrix Reimprinting. I took each of his classes several times. In 2019, I joined a business community called Thrive Academy in Santa Cruz. It's a very supportive community. Studying these complementary methods helped me with the burnout from nursing. Mastering a whole new body of knowledge is really exciting for me.

In the last twenty-seven years of my career, I worked in emergency rooms. Most of my career was in critical care. I worked ten years in coronary care, and then I did six years of floating the floors and in ICU, CCU. I worked a year and a half in obstetrical recovery. And then I went to the ER.

What has been the most challenging aspect of your career in general?

I've always had a problem with boundaries, being able to say no. And of course, in most jobs, you don't have a lot of options to say no. I couldn't say, "I don't want that assignment." In my last job, I had no choice whatsoever, as far as what patient assignments I had. That was just the way that job was set up.

There were times when I thought, I can't stand this anymore, so I'd change areas, and that helped; I'd get to learn something new. And I recognized that yes, I want to have a private coaching practice, but nursing was my profession. I was just going to work and getting paid for it, which was easy, but now being an entrepreneur is a whole different ballgame. I've noticed over the past eight years, since retiring from nursing, there's a mindset shift that has to happen. I was an employee for my entire career. And to go from employee to entrepreneur is an evolution.

Do you find the nursing profession stressful? How do you cope with the stress?

It wasn't until I retired that I recognized I'd been carrying the weight of life-and-death responsibility on my shoulders. Even when I was off, I worried about the little mistakes I made here or the bigger mistake I made over there. And I did not realize I carried that until I was out of the profession. And in the ER, being pulled in different directions and not being able to complete something was frustrating.

Studying and learning new things helped me with stress and burnout. I worked full time in nursing for a while and then went to 0.8, and then went to a 0.6. During my last job, I'd worked nights, and it was exhausting. I didn't have enough energy left over to have a private practice. I'd try to remember to practice self-care to handle stress. I'm better now than I was at remembering to use the tools I'd learned to self-regulate. Because I'm psychic, I get pulled off-balance easily; that's another example of me not setting good boundaries.

Many of us aren't raised by parents who know how to self-regulate. So, when you're expected to self-regulate, it takes learning, and it's a life-long process.

Have there been times you didn't practice self-care when you knew you needed to?

At first, I didn't even know about self-care. Instead, the phrase used was "get a hold of yourself." But I didn't know how. Learning EFT has made a huge difference for me. I now can address the uncomfortable feelings I have and move them out of my body. Emotional acupressure is such a helpful tool.

What words or ideas would you offer to help nurses in their career that you wish you'd known?

Number one: Take your breaks. Don't work through breaks and don't stay after work to finish your charting off the clock. With electronic charting now, it's harder to do that. But don't give the workplace time that's not paid for. Charting is part of the job. And if you can't chart as you go, and you must do it afterward, be sure you charge hours for it. Because too much overtime is the only thing that gets hospitals to add more staff. And that's what's needed.

Nurses are a population of caretakers and helpers who won't just walk away from patients. They're being taken advantage of, which is a setup for burnout.

Many of the younger people have more hutzpah than I ever did as a child who grew up in the 1950s. Women have much more of a voice now than they used to have. Boundaries have to be learned. The kids whose "no" is not honored are the ones that have to learn they have a right to say that. When they're asked to take on one extra patient, it's important to say, "I'm full. I have enough to do right here. I can't do that right now," or say, "No, I can't work five extra shifts this week." If you're tired, you're going to miss cues from your patients. You might miss information or get confused. So, rest is a vital ingredient in being a good nurse. And you do have the right to have a good time.

Before I retired, I was chosen as a juror on a stressful three-week trial. The jury met Monday through Friday, and I worked nights Thursday through Sunday. I only took off a couple of Thursdays, and I didn't ask off for any extra days, even though I was on this jury, which I realize now was silly.

During the last week of the trial, we were released from jury duty for Martin Luther King Day because the court was closed. My head nurse left a message for me, asking me to lead a skills-day session on Thursday because I was off. I said, "It's my only day off this week." She kept asking, but I was able to stand firm because I'd only had four days off in three weeks.

What has been the most rewarding aspect of your nursing career?

I enjoyed the patient contact. Not all of it, but most of it. I enjoyed teaching people, and especially in the ER, I gave excellent discharge instructions; if somebody had a broken leg, I taught them the best ways to handle that at home while thinking about everything they do, because nothing will be automatic since they have an injury or an illness interfering with their regular routine. I think the most rewarding part of my nursing career was teaching and then seeing when my patients understood.

Teaching is a natural skill for me. In my last job, I learned Spanish because we had a lot of Hispanic people who would come to the ER. For example, when a child had an ear infection, and Dad, who was home from his two jobs, bundled the whole family into the car to come to the ER for the night, being able to communicate with them was very satisfying.

I was extremely detailed when giving parents instructions on how to dose with Tylenol and ibuprofen for kids with fevers. I'd write out a schedule and calculate the dose for them, then explain why I was doing it that way so they can self-manage at home.

Is there anything else you'd like to share with nurses that could make their lives better?

When nurses are so depleted because they haven't been able to say no, they need to take a break before their body insists on a break—before they injure themselves or get sick. The body will say, "That's enough."

If they find themselves crying on the way to work, that's a sign that maybe they need to do something different. The money and benefits are tough to give up. And it's hard to change jobs and give up your seniority. But if you dread going to work, if you cry on the way to work, if you don't want to do it anymore, or if you can't find any joy in it, then it's time for a change—honor that.

Burnout is an emotional pain. When you don't care anymore or when you get to the point where you just can't deal with other people's pain anymore, you go numb. That doesn't help anybody. It doesn't help you, and it doesn't help your patients. Take care of yourself. You matter!

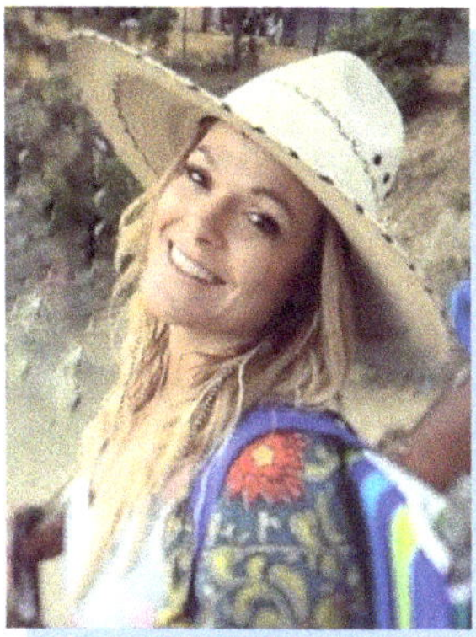

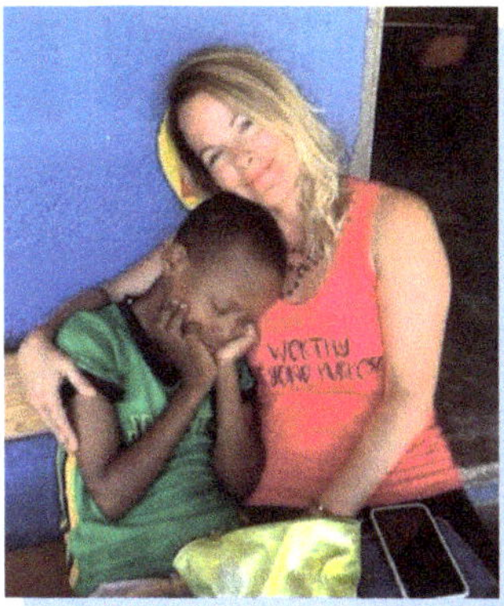

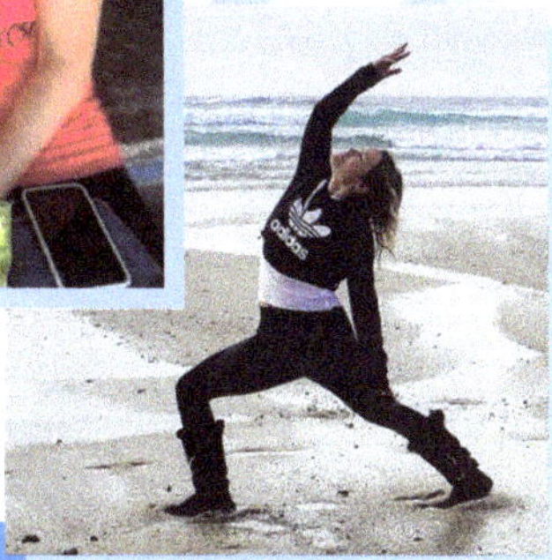

Jessica Brown, RN, RYT

California

What made you decide to become a nurse? Was there someone or an event that influenced you?

Honestly, I found myself pregnant at a young age and knew I needed to make a living to support us both as a single mother. That being said, I'm a highly compassionate human, and nursing is where I was meant to begin my journey/career.

Tell me about your nursing career, such as where you have practiced, what types of facilities you've served in, and how long you have served as a nurse.

I've been a nurse for nineteen years. I thought I wanted to work in the OR, but after one year, I realized it wasn't for me. After that, I did one year in a step-down/telemetry unit and then to trauma SICU. I absolutely loved this job and worked with the most amazing team ever. I learned so much and felt great when helping people and seeing them recover. Of course, there were many sad and depressing cases as well.

I worked in MICU, which I didn't care for because these patients rarely get better, and there are many repeat customers. I started traveling and worked in many different departments. I would say the ER was fun and social but carried the most stress. Working in big cities was always a battle, and sometimes, I'd go to a smaller rural hospital in the middle of nowhere to regroup.

What has been the most challenging aspect of your career in general?

There's a sick culture among nurses: bullying. Possibly because it's such a stressful job, but I've encountered many rude and nasty coworkers in my day. I always stand for justice and learned to have strong boundaries over the years. If I ever witness other nurses coming down on "baby" nurses, I always stick up for them. Especially ER and ICU nurses, where bullying seems to be an ongoing battle. I've worked both, so I see where it stems from.

Do you find the nursing profession stressful? How do you cope with the stress?

Yes. It's an extremely stressful job. Between the family members' abuse, coworkers, and doctors, it's pretty unbearable. As you may be able to tell, I'm burned out. If I could take care of ailing patients and just be compassionate and heartfelt, that would be perfect. Unfortunately, the system doesn't allow it.

From 2004-2017, I coped with stress with drugs and alcohol. I broke my back in 2003, and this was the beginning of my fourteen-year opiate addiction battle. Shortly after, I struggled with a broken heart, and the doctor gave me Xanax. Add that to the opiates, and it was a BIG battle.

In 2017, I changed my life through prayer, yoga, meditation, 12-steps, and a multitude of inner work, mostly connecting to myself and learning to love myself. I have worked with family constellations, ancestral healing, and I'm a yoga and meditation teacher now. And I have a non-profit that teaches mindfulness to children.[3] I found getting sober very difficult as a nurse, but by the grace of God—I did it!!

How has the COVID-19 pandemic affected your work?

I was working in Los Angeles and on the verge of quitting nursing altogether because of the stress. Right when COVID-19 hit in March, I had a difficult experience with getting PPE for a possible COVID-19 patient. I quit after that day per my husband's order (he was sick of my constant misery). I started teaching yoga and meditation here and there and using my savings. I took a travel assignment in Hawaii in a tiny town in the middle of nowhere, and it's been four months of pure bliss. I have many friends that have horrible experiences, and I pray for them daily. A few have contracted COVID-19 and recovered also.

Have there been times you didn't practice self-care when you knew you needed to?

Yes, all the years I was numbing out. If I got stressed, I took a pill.

If I didn't have a connection to myself and God, I could never do this job sober. I love caring for sick people, but it isn't easy to do this in the healthcare system.

What words or ideas would you offer to help nurses in their career that you wish you'd known?

I have a morning ritual/practice that saves me.

I pray and meditate and practice yoga in the morning. If I'm short on time, then my yoga is short and sweet, but prayer and meditation are essential. Honestly, I pray throughout the day. I practice Reiki on myself after work and usually listen to a guided meditation before sleeping. I always create a bubble of golden light around me for protection before I walk in a hospital. I bring essential oils like lavender and sage. I carry crystals in my pocket for protection also.

What has been the most rewarding aspect of your nursing career?

I took care of a gentleman who was in a head-on collision and had multiple injuries and was in a coma for three months. I got very close with his wife during their time in ICU, where she always requested me as his nurse. One day while I was assessing him at the beginning of my shift, he awoke from his coma. It was so amazing to witness. He left for rehab a month or so later.

His daughter got married two years later, and I was invited to the wedding. That was the first time we met in person, and he thanked me for everything.

Is there anything else you'd like to share with nurses that could make their lives better?

Be kind … but have strong boundaries! Protect your energy and physical well-being! Drink more water and less coffee! Don't get addicted to making money. Taking care of yourself and your own family is the most important thing. I've seen so many nurses working so much overtime to buy more "things." Your health and time are way more important than money and things!!!

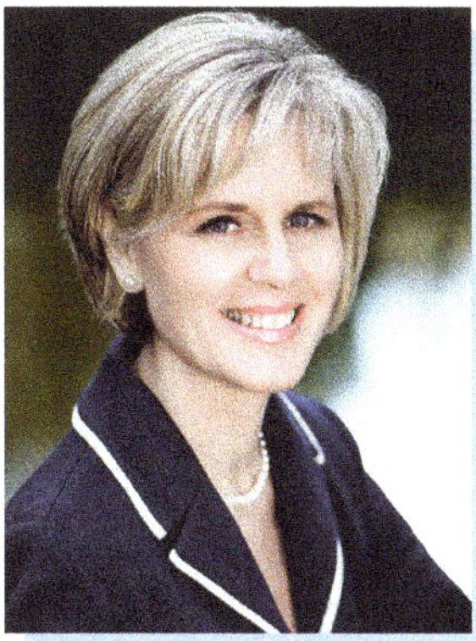

Pamela McDonald, PNP, FNP

California

What made you decide to become a nurse? Was there someone or an event that influenced you?

As a fourteen-year-old in England, we had to decide what we wanted to become and then worked for our exams. After exploring the world of nursing, I decided it would be a wonderful profession to be in. I loved everything about it, from the smell of a hospital to the uniform, including that white starched apron, the blue belt with the shining buckle, and the hats. I was going to become a nurse, and I was so excited once I made the decision.

Tell me about your nursing career, such as where you have practiced, what types of facilities you've served in, and how long you have served as a nurse.

I began my nursing education at the Royal Hospital of St. Bartholomew's right in the center of London, England.

In 1980, I moved to California and became a volunteer at the University of California in San Francisco. Then I worked for a registry in San Francisco and worked in all the San Francisco hospitals for about two years.

I moved to the East Bay and worked in an oncology unit, where I had an experience with a patient diagnosed with breast cancer. I helped her into the shower after she ate breakfast. While she was in the shower, I was going to strip her bed and make it all nice and clean and fresh so she could rest comfortably. As I returned from collecting her fresh linens, the hall shower door opened up, and she came out crying. She put her hands up to the sky and said, "God, why do I have breast cancer?" and then fell to the floor and sobbed.

That question she asked got me to ask the question also—and what kept coming up was what we eat. How we manage this body can cause cancer to become turned on. My question was, well, if smoking causes cancer, what else could be causing it? Is it the food we eat, the fluids we drink, the air or smoke we breathe? And what about the exercise and energy we put out? Are we managing our energy in our bodies?

All these questions kept coming up. Within a few months, I had gone to the hospital administration and started an employee exercise program. It quickly moved into a community wellness program with Covert Bailey and the national center for health promotion. The wellness center is still open today.

Then I moved to Santa Barbara and became the director of health education at Sansom Medical Center. Afterward, I worked in labor and delivery, and then I went back to school to become a nurse practitioner.

Because of my experience in labor and delivery, nursery, OR, and Level II newborn ICU, I became a women's health nurse practitioner. I then completed the adult primary care nurse practitioner program. I went to UCLA and completed the first assistant surgery program and completed my pediatric nurse practitioner program and family nurse practitioner program. I opened my medical practice in 2003, and it is still open today.[4]

In 2005, I completed a two-year fellowship at the Center for Integrative Medicine at the College of Medicine at the University of

Arizona and became a faculty member with Dr. Andrew Weil, Dr. Victoria Maizes, and Fredi Kronenberg, PhD.

What has been the most challenging aspect of your career in general?

The most challenging aspect of my career is access and reimbursement of care, other than allopathic medicine. Integrative medicine has been formally established for over twenty-five years now. Over 100 medical schools have some integrative medicine in their curriculum, but insurance companies do not allow time and reimbursement for this type of medicine. Insurance companies will pay for a procedure, a pill, or surgery, but they will generally not pay for time with a patient. It's an uphill battle. What about teaching a patient about botanical medicine, nutritional medicine, sports medicine, mind-body medicine; all these things are not supported and are much less expensive than an expensive medication or surgery. The problem is that a pill or surgery is used 100 percent of the time when they should be used 20–25 percent of the time.

Do you find the nursing profession stressful? How do you cope with the stress?

I believe that I've created a practice where the stress is relatively low.

Charting is a stressor, and so is getting paid by the insurance company, but other than that, there's relatively low stress.

How has the COVID-19 pandemic affected your work?

I've transitioned well with COVID-19, as I'm able to take care of my patients via telemedicine. I'm also seeing that when a patient has changed their diet and exercise and are taking care of their health, they're not getting sick. An example is when I had a family who had three children, one at college and two at home. Mom and dad followed the APO E gene diet, and their oldest child got COVID-19, and she was very sick. She came home and was being cared for by the mom mostly, but everyone was exposed to the virus; however, the level of symptoms was all different depending on how they followed their anti-inflammatory APO E diet. The college student did NOT follow the APO E diet, but the mom and dad did. The college student got COVID-19, and even though the mom and dad were exposed, they didn't have the symptoms of the virus.

Have there been times you didn't practice self-care when you knew you needed to?

The only time I didn't focus on taking care of myself was when I was opening my medical practice. I was burning the candle at both ends, and my husband encouraged me to see someone, and he was right as usual.

But what I learned was amazing. I discovered why I was doing what I was doing in my work, so it was highly beneficial for me.

What words or ideas would you offer to help nurses in their career that you wish you'd known?

I think all nurses need to take care of themselves.

All nurses should get their APO E gene tested.

Also, I believe that all nurses could benefit from a specific type of daily yoga, especially a practice called Inner Engineering.

What has been the most rewarding aspect of your nursing career?

The most rewarding part of my work has been creating the APO E gene program. It has shown me that patients can get better if given a chance based on the right diet for the person's APO E gene.

Is there anything else you'd like to share with nurses that could make their lives better?

I think integrative medicine is the NEW medicine and more nurses need to learn how to integrate it into their lives. It's not that difficult.

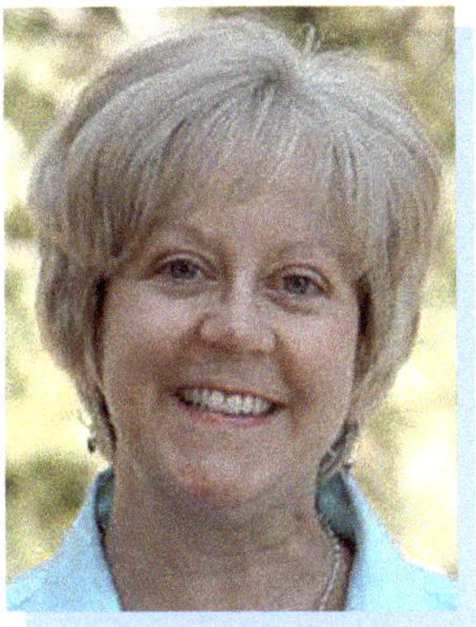

Mary Ann Osborne, DNP, RN, FNP-BC

Colorado

What made you decide to become a nurse? Was there someone or an event that influenced you?

When I was seven years old, I was in an accident, where a tractor ran completely over me. Yes, the BIG wheel of the tractor. I was wearing a new outfit, which was white with blue trim, and the tire tread marks went all the way up my back. I didn't suffer any broken bones; however, I did have intense muscle injury, and a public health nurse came to our home and did physical therapy several times a week and taught me how to walk again! I was so in "awe" of her and it was such a significant event.

Then after I recovered, one day I went with my parents to see my aunt at her jobsite, and when she walked out to meet us, she was in a crisp, white uniform with her nursing hat, and I was mesmerized. I believe these two events impressed upon me to decide that I wanted to be a nurse and help others.

Tell me about your nursing career, such as where you have practiced, what types of facilities you've served in, and how long you have served as a nurse.

I graduated with my BSN in 1979 and went back to my North Carolina hometown and worked for several years in our local hospital. Then I decided that I wanted to travel and "see the world," and I joined the Army Nurse Corps. My initial assignment was in Colorado, and I worked in an orthopedic/neurological unit and then became head nurse of a medicine unit.

I then decided to apply to the army's adult medical/surgical nurse practitioner program, and upon graduation in 1986, I was once again stationed in Colorado at Fort Carson. This was a wonderful experience.

From there, I went back to school to get a master's degree as a family nurse practitioner and then had assignments in Germany, Kansas, Virginia, and Washington State. I held nurse practitioner and administrative positions in army community hospitals and medical centers. I was the first army nurse to manage a team, which oversaw all aspects of outpatient medicine, and thus was in charge of all personnel to include physicians.

My last army assignment was as the section chief for all outpatient clinics and the emergency room of a major army medical center. At the end of my army career, I went back to school. I was the first nurse practitioner to graduate from the Fellowship in Integrative Medicine at the University of Arizona in 2003.

I retired with the rank of Lieutenant Colonel and twenty-one years of service from the army in 2003. Then I moved back to Colorado and worked with several like-minded practitioners in private practice and in public health. In 2013, I opened my own integrative nurse practitioner practice[5] and am so happy I took this step. I love having my own practice and providing care in the way I feel everyone should be offered care, including teaching others about self-care and holistic/integrative ways of healing and health promotion.

What has been the most challenging aspect of your career in general?

Taking care of myself with the demands of my career. I wish self-care had been taught in my nursing programs. While serving in the army, there were physical fitness requirements, and I had to pass my physical training (PT) test; however, while most of those serving in the military have PT as part of their daily job, when working in nursing, you don't have this opportunity. You must find the time outside of your shift or clinic duty for physical fitness (just like all nurses). As I've gotten older and have had more education and experience, I see the importance of caring for oneself in order to care for others.

I'm also grateful that I always listened to my intuition. I know that my patients have benefited from my courage to speak up or call for help when I "knew" something was wrong or "wasn't right" with my patient. In my clinic setting, information often shows up to me a few days before seeing a client who happens to need this information. It has been challenging not to ignore this—because it's not as acceptable in our culture and profession. But it's important to connect to this sense that we all carry and have access to.

Do you find the nursing profession stressful? How do you cope with the stress?

Nursing is a stressful profession. There's a lot of pressure placed on nurses in our current disease management for-profit system, and we're pushed to do our jobs with less time. That's one reason I decided to start my practice. However, being a business owner is also stressful. I started meditating in 2001, and it's the best decision I've ever made for myself. It has greatly increased the serenity in my life.

How has the COVID-19 pandemic affected your work?

COVID-19 has impacted my life and practice. I'm lucky that since I have my own practice, it was easier for me to follow the guidelines from the Colorado Department of Health. I'm very grateful they have provided clear guidelines.

Initially, I was fearful that my business might not survive as demand dropped a great deal. I'm using predominantly telehealth and work with my clients to improve their immune systems with positive lifestyle changes, supplements, and improved management of any chronic disease. Now is the time for everyone to learn how to live in a way that lowers their inflammation, and thus, decrease the risk of getting COVID-19. I do continue to see some clients in person, and it is different with masks, distance, and minimal exams, and no hugging.

While serving in the US Army, we often discussed and prepared for the next pandemic. So, it's possible that, mentally, I was better prepared and not shocked this happened. We've always known it would happen but just not *when* it would happen. It's important to remember that it will not last forever. It is also important to reflect on what we would like to keep from our lifestyle changes that the COVID-19 experience has offered. For me, I was saying "Yes" to too many things and traveling away from home too often. It's helped me to see that I was yearning for a slower, simpler life, and I desire to stay connected with those people, pets, and nature that bring joy into each day.

Have there been times you didn't practice self-care when you knew you needed to?

Absolutely. I've had times in my life when other life stressors interfered with my ability to continue self-care. My husband has had cancer twice and aseptic meningitis, and my long-time childhood friend died from a long and slow neurological degenerative disease. Those are just a few examples of ten consecutive years of varying loss. Those events not only take your time but also your energy at a core level. I survived this with my meditation practice and support from colleagues, friends, and family.

What words or ideas would you offer to help nurses in their career that you wish you'd known?

First, take care of yourself! It will appear that you don't have time for self-care; however, if you make the time for movement, eating well, and time for reflection, you'll have more energy for yourself and others.

In addition, I recommend some type of mind-body practice that you use regularly. The mind and body are not separate; they're only separate when we say the words. You can tap into the body's innate healing ability and use it for yourself.

Don't hesitate to ask for help.

Continue to learn and pay attention to what interests you and follow your intuition.

What has been the most rewarding aspect of your nursing career?

The most rewarding aspect of my career is that I fell in love with my profession. Being with people in the worst moments of their lives and the best moments of their lives is a privilege. Nurses are able to be with our patients and their families at these moments. Actively listening to their stories and really "being present" with them in the moment. Assisting clients to find their path to healing and wellness and/or assisting them on their path to transitioning in death. All of those moments have been rewarding. Also, making lifelong friends with my nursing colleagues has been one of the greatest rewards of choosing nursing as my profession.

Is there anything else you'd like to share with nurses that could make their lives better?

I think one of the most important skills you can learn and cultivate for yourself and your nursing practice is to learn to "be present" during the moments of your life. This doesn't come naturally to our active thinking brains. Take a class or find a mentor but cultivate mindful awareness in your life. You are not the only one whose thoughts are going in all directions. You can cultivate an ability to have an awareness of your thoughts and bring yourself back to the present moment. This is where happiness lives.

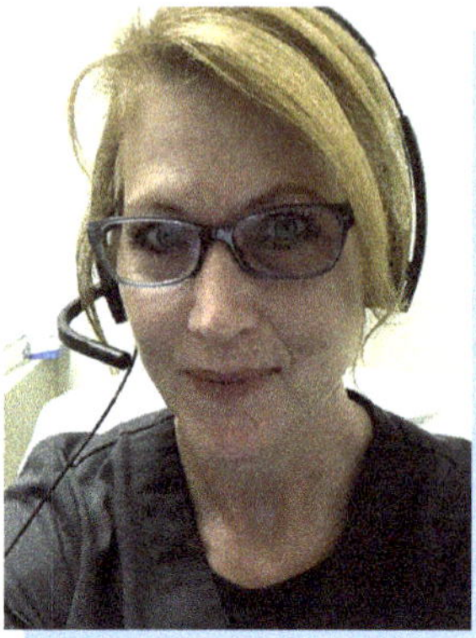

Jennifer, APRN

Florida

What made you decide to become a nurse? Was there someone or an event that influenced you?

It was just a calling; I love helping people. My mother was my strongest influence in choosing this profession. My maternal grandmother was a nurse too. I guess it's in the blood.

Tell me about your nursing career, such as where you have practiced, what types of facilities you've served in, and how long you have served as a nurse.

I've been an RN since 1991, and I've been a nurse practitioner since 2010. As an RN, I have worked in the hospital in medical/surgical, pediatrics, pediatric ER, pediatric ICU, PACU/preop, mom/baby, labor and delivery (dabbled a little), special care nursery, and NICU. As an RN outpatient, I've worked in home health as a nurse case manager, home health coordinator, and PACU in a surgery center. I've been a charge nurse, supervisor, nurse educator, and staff nurse.

As a nurse practitioner, I've done infectious disease specialty, family practice/primary care, urgent care/occupational health, and a little ortho. Currently, I'm trapped in telemedicine for sick employees, hoping someday once COVID-19 is gone, we will go back to an urgent care setting.

What has been the most challenging aspect of your career in general?

Dealing with the COVID-19 pandemic. Balancing grad school, a full-time job, and parenting. I survived it! When working in PICU, the death of a child. I can still remember each child.

Do you find the nursing profession stressful? How do you cope with the stress?

Yes. There are good days and bad days. I exercise to destress and make sure there's a separation of work and home (not so much during COVID-19). Work kind of swallows everything.

How has the COVID-19 pandemic affected your work?

This has been the craziest few months of my nursing career. First, long hours, PPE equipment shortages (reusing PPE all day that you would normally throw away after one use), protocols for COVID-19 changing every few days, going to virtual visits, and getting exposed to the virus, followed by being quarantined. Now there are health system financial problems with people getting laid off and furloughed. There's no end in sight, just fatigue from this grind.

I work in an employee health clinic, which is like an urgent care and free clinic for our employees only, so I deal with sick and stressed out employees all day. I can see the strain and fatigue in the frontline workers. I see the fear when I tell an employee they are COVID-19 positive. I could go on and on. I have gone from seeing patients in person to telemedicine, and I'm told this will carry into next year.

There are things I see administration doing that I think are wrong. I don't think we are appreciated. What I do see is we're all easily dispensable if the healthcare system's finances don't improve.

Have there been times you didn't practice self-care when you knew you needed to?

Yes, a lot recently. I'm just overwhelmed by COVID-19.

What words or ideas would you offer to help nurses in their career that you wish you'd known?

Patience. Take a deep breath when you feel overwhelmed. Ask for help. Be a team player. Wear support stockings! LOL.

What has been the most rewarding aspect of your nursing career?

Helping people.

Is there anything else you'd like to share with nurses that could make their lives better?

Continue your education.

MORGAN, DNP, ARNP

Iowa

What made you decide to become a nurse? Was there someone or an event that influenced you?

I first became interested in nursing while watching hospice nurses care for a family member when I was a child. From there, I became more interested in human sciences and then shifted my educational goals toward something in the healthcare setting. In high school, I got my CNA and worked in my rural Iowa community nursing home.

Tell me about your nursing career, such as where you have practiced, what types of facilities you've served in, and how long you have served as a nurse.

I knew I wanted to be part of the healthcare team from a young age. Growing up in a rural setting, this is often an underserved population, and I wanted to ultimately transition back into the small-town health-care setting if able. I looked into medical school, PA, and ultimately with my personal goals, nursing was the perfect fit.

I started with my four-year degree but always knew that I would want to further my education. I graduated with my BSN and started working in a rural hospital. Eventually, I wanted to end up in a small hospital, but I needed more experience. To gain additional experience I moved to a more urban setting (Des Moines) to get better experience on a cardiac telemetry floor.

Fortunately, I was accepted to the University of Iowa Doctorate of Nursing Practice's family practice program. While starting the graduate program, I transitioned to pediatric hematology/oncology nursing at the University of Iowa to get pediatric experience.

Upon completion of my program, I had a difficult time finding a primary care position. Eventually, I started in pain management in an urban setting, which was an eye-opening experience. Pain management is not generally a popular specialty, but I found it both challenging and rewarding.

Fortunately, an opportunity opened in a hospitalist role at a critical access hospital. Rural health care also has its own set of challenges and experiences.

What has been the most challenging aspect of your career in general?

Health care is challenging in general, from staying on top of the latest research, technology, and medications, to keeping up to date with all the latest insurance and Medicare guidelines.

Now that I'm working in a rural community, I'm experiencing various issues that I hadn't even thought of before. Access to specialties in these areas is becoming an ever-present problem. Provider retention is becoming a huge topic of discussion. Specialists are hard to come by. How can these small towns possibly recruit, let alone compete, with the more urban settings?

Outpatient specialty clinics are a helpful resource, but these are often only once a month. When we have someone acutely admitted to the hospital, often, recommendations are made through an over-the-phone consultation with a follow-up outpatient. Then there's another problem: access/transportation issues for patients trying to get to these appointments. With increasing technology, telehealth is becoming a possible answer—but that comes with an added expense as well.

There are no easy answers, but hopefully, as more of these issues are brought to light, there will be better opportunities for better access to healthcare in the future.

Do you find the nursing profession stressful? How do you cope with the stress?

Nursing is a very stressful position. We see people at their best and their worst. It's hard not to internalize what we see and do when we're naturally an empathetic profession. With all the HIPPA guidelines in place to protect HPI, it also creates a barrier to healthcare workers when we need to vent or de-stress, because we're not supposed to talk about what happened during our shift.

Being in a more leadership position as a nurse practitioner, I tend to seek out the nursing staff after a stressful situation to check in on them emotionally and mentally. By openly discussing situations after they happen, it not only helps me cope, but I also think it has helped others.

Have there been times you didn't practice self-care when you knew you needed to?

Early on in graduate school, when I was working while going to school, I wasn't able to take care of myself as much as I should have. Ultimately, I decided that I needed to cut back at work and went part time. This extra time was not necessarily put toward only studying, but also spending time with family and friends, which I desperately needed.

What words or ideas would you offer to help nurses in their career that you wish you'd known?

I often ask the nurses I work with, "If you were a patient, what advice would you give them?" Often, we (as nurses) are so used to taking care of others that we often neglect ourselves. By thinking of ourselves as the patients, it helps shift our way of thinking. Often, we see the caregiver-role strain in family members who are constantly taking care of loved ones. Well, nursing is very similar. We need to take time to care for ourselves.

What has been the most rewarding aspect of your nursing career?

Patient care, and ultimately watching people heal and improve. It's amazing to see healthcare evidence-based practices work in real time and take people from the brink of death back to their baseline.

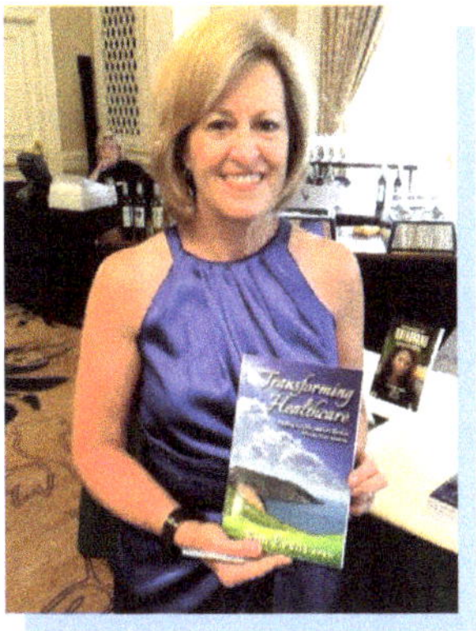

Kim Evans, APRN, CNS-BC, AHN-BC, CNAT

Kentucky

What made you decide to become a nurse? Was there someone or an event that influenced you?

My aunt, who is five years older than me, is an X-ray technician. I wanted to follow in her footsteps. However, she convinced me that there were many more opportunities in healthcare if I became a nurse. I took her advice and am so glad I did!

Tell me about your nursing career, such as where you have practiced, what types of facilities you've served in, and how long you have served as a nurse.

I've always had a passion for helping people heal. I became a registered nurse in 1977. I worked in critical care units, such as respiratory intensive care (including being the head nurse), coronary care, surgical intensive care, emergency departments, and post-anesthesia care.

In 1993, I attended a conference called "Healing the Healer Within" (presented by Barbara Dossey, Cathy Guzetta, and Chris Kessler), which literally changed my life. It opened my eyes to a whole new world of holistic nursing and healing the whole person—body, mind, and spirit. I applied much of this whole-person approach to my work as a critical care specialist. We utilized music therapy, touch therapy, massage, and guided imagery with patients for pain control, stress reduction, and to enhance overall well-being.

I resigned from my critical care Clinical Nurse Specialist position in August 1996 and I completed the two-year certificate program in Amma therapy, a form of acupressure based on Traditional Chinese Medicine taught by Anneke Young, a protégé of Mrs. Tina Sohn.

In 1997, I started my practice offering Amma therapy and a holistic nursing assessment. In 2000, I met three other practitioners (Dr. Slava Paskovich, a physician from Ukraine; Eddie Campomonas, a physical therapist; and Amber Stone, a PT assistant who was trained in massage, cranial sacral therapy, and strain/counter-strain techniques). They were interested in creating an integrative medicine center, and together, we started the Institute for Integrative Medicine.[6] We worked together for three years.

Life events ensued, and Dr. Paskovich and Eddie Campomonas both relocated to different areas of the country. I continued as the sole owner of the Institute for Integrative Medicine.

In June 2003, while meditating and contemplating on how to continue my vision to change the healthcare system, I dreamed of writing a book on transforming healthcare. I knew I needed a publishing class and I wanted to see a hospital in Hawaii that I had heard about and knew was the epitome of how future hospitals should be designed and managed.

In October 2003, my husband and I attended the Integrative Medicine Cardiology Conference cosponsored by the North Hawaii Community Hospital. It was surreal. Only 108 people attended; however, they were the powerhouses in integrative medicine. Dr. Dean Ornish, Dr. Andrew Weil, Dr. Robert Superko, Dr. Mimi Guarneri, and Dr. David Eisenberg were some of the conference attendees.

On the second day of the conference, I met an exceptional nurse practitioner, Pam McDonald. We immediately connected and have become life-long friends/colleagues. We knew that our passions and visions were similar, and we were both committed to change cardiovascular care and the overall health of Americans. My practice expanded to become the Kentucky site for doing APO E gene testing.

My passion for holistic nursing and integrative medicine continued to expand. I enrolled in the University of Arizona Program for Integrative Medicine, which is the premier education in the country for integrative medicine. The Fellowship provided an extraordinary opportunity to study with Dr. Andrew Weil, Dr. Tieraona Low Dog, and Dr. Victoria Maizes. I completed the Fellowship in December 2006.

Also, in 2006, along with several committed nurses, we revived the Kentucky Holistic Nurses Association (KHNA).

We grew and expanded our services, and on November 1, 2010, we moved to our current office location. It took one year to find the ideal space, location, and practitioners. We are very excited to be together, help each other be as healthy as possible, and forward the science of holistic healing and integrative medicine. I am privileged to work with outstanding, dedicated practitioners.

What has been the most challenging aspect of your career in general?

The most challenging aspect has been to practice true "health care" based on wellness and disease prevention in a system rooted in disease-care and profit margins. The current disease-care system expands as it keeps people sick and diseased. It's the antithesis of what our goals are when helping people achieve their optimal health of mind, body, and spirit.

As my desire to heal the whole person grew, my frustration with the hospital system increased. I found that the system was NOT patient- and family-centered. One example is the fact that we would awaken patients at 4:30 or 5:00 AM to draw blood or do an X-ray so these results could be available when the physician made rounds at 7:00 AM. This remains a common practice today in most healthcare facilities.

Do you find the nursing profession stressful? How do you cope with the stress?

I love being a nurse and having my own clinic. It has required a lot of work and is stressful at times. However, my clinic is filled with stress management providers. I'm attentive to my own self-care with meditation, daily exercise, and prayer. I also have regular chiropractic visits, pedicures, Havening sessions, and occasional massage therapy.

How has the COVID-19 pandemic affected your work?

We have been open every day during the COVID-19 pandemic. We've supported people by helping them keep their immune systems healthy with vitamins and supplements. We've answered continuing calls about symptom management, COVID-19 exposures, and testing options. Our patient visits never stopped. For the first six to eight weeks, all of our patient visits were held via telemedicine Zoom sessions. Currently, we are doing about 50 percent in-office visits with all suggested precautions and 50 percent telemedicine sessions.

Have there been times you didn't practice self-care when you knew you needed to?

My Achilles' heel is not getting enough sleep. But during this COVID-19 pandemic, despite being very busy, we've increased our exercise, which has boosted our self-care practice.

What words or ideas would you offer to help nurses in their career that you wish you'd known?

Now is the time for nurses to thrive. We have so many opportunities. The COVID-19 has blatantly revealed problems in our disease-care system. People realize the value of wellness strategies and disease prevention, which is all NURSING! Let the medical professionals carry out disease care. Let nurses take over health and well-being. This is how we can transform healthcare.

What has been the most rewarding aspect of your nursing career?

Having my practice and being able to spend time with patients to truly help them transform their health of mind, body, and spirit.

Is there anything else you'd like to share with nurses that could make their lives better?

Let's heal ourselves, and then we can heal healthcare. Let's create a camaraderie in nursing of "I've Got Your Back" and support each other to transform nursing and healthcare completely.

Eat healthily, exercise regularly, and practice daily prayer/meditation/Inner Engineering.

I was able to publish my book, *Transforming Healthcare: Healing You, Me and Our Broken Disease-Care System.*[7] I know that nurses are at a pivotal moment in transforming healthcare. It begins with transforming ourselves. Let's transform healthcare by transforming nursing.

Florence Nightingale predicted it would take 200 years to transform healthcare. Now is the time!!

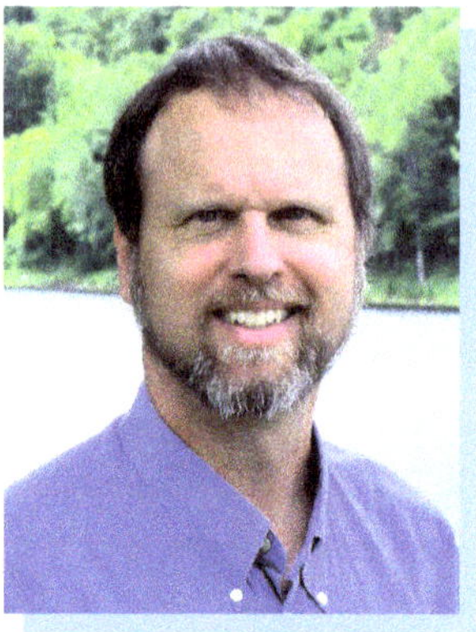

Tom Bartol, NP

Maine

What made you decide to become a nurse? Was there someone or an event that influenced you?

It was my senior year in high school, many years ago. I was supposed to be an engineer but had decided math wasn't for me. Everyone in my family went to college, so I felt pressure to go but had no idea what I wanted to do.

I had an excellent anatomy and physiology teacher in high school, who was also a rough and tough football coach, but I really liked learning about the human body. There was an opportunity to take an Emergency Medical Technician class at age sixteen. I enjoyed volunteering in the emergency room, so I decided to become a nurse. It was a last-minute decision without a lot more thought, but it worked out well.

Tell me about your nursing career, such as where you have practiced, what types of facilities you've served in, and how long you have served as a nurse.

I took paramedic training during my first year of nursing school and worked in EMS and liked it. I also worked as an aide in the emergency room. But after graduation from nursing school, I decided to do at least a year of medical/surgical nursing to really know what nursing was all about. I did that, and then the hospital where I worked started an air ambulance program. As a nurse and paramedic, despite my lack of ER experience, they accepted me.

I worked the air ambulance and ER for three years. It was exciting, and I loved the work, but one day, I realized it wasn't making a lot of difference. People survived, they lived, but, for many, there wasn't much "life" ahead after head injuries and spinal cord injuries. It seemed like I wasn't making the difference I wanted to make.

I thought I would go to Africa and do some volunteer nursing work and ended up volunteering in Nome, Alaska, for three years. I worked at an eighteen-bed hospital. On night shift, there were three people in the hospital, two nurses and a janitor. We answered the phones, were security, housekeeping, ER, OB, and everything. We even had a six-bed nursing home. I learned to change diapers and deliver babies and everything from CCU to pediatrics. It was a tremendous experience.

Three years later, I rode my bike home from Alaska and then went on to Sierra Leone, West Africa, to do volunteer work there. I worked in a mission hospital, teaching nursing students. At the time, nursing students mostly ran the hospital, along with sharpening and sterilizing needles, washing and sterilizing surgical gloves, and giving patient care. It was an eye-opening experience of what can be, and of people caring.

I left Sierra Leone when the civil war started in that country and eventually found my way back to the United States. I had decided to go back to school to become a nurse practitioner but because I had been living out of the country and wasn't a resident of any state, I didn't meet any college residency requirements. So I decided to go to El Paso, Texas, and do volunteer work at a refugee shelter. I learned to speak Spanish and to work in a shelter and also helped start healthcare for the homeless in El Paso—since undocumented people only had the ER for their health care.

After nine months of living and working at the refugee shelter as a volunteer, I moved to Seattle, Washington, to begin my training as a nurse practitioner at the University of Washington (UW).

I had an excellent education at UW and made many friends. I graduated in 1994 with my master's degree and moved to Okanogan, Washington, to do a Migrant Health Fellowship. I worked at a community health center with the migrant apple pickers and learned a lot while putting the Spanish I learned in El Paso to good use.

When the fellowship ended, I moved to Kansas City, Missouri, and worked for two years in a community health center serving the Hispanic population. I focused half of my time on family practice and the other half developing a diabetes program for the patients at the health center. At this time, I was asked to give a talk on diabetes at the University of Missouri at Kansas City, and it began a new phase in my career of speaking and writing. I began speaking around the country on diabetes and then on many other subjects as well as writing chapters for books and articles for publication on a variety of topics.

Two years later, I was laid off from the community health center. There was a private clinic in a poor section of town, just blocks from where I lived, and I dropped off my résumé there with a cover letter. Within hours, I had a job.

The physician owner had just lost a physician and was desperate for help. She had never worked with NPs but was willing to try and learn. This became one of the best jobs of my life. We worked together in this inner-city clinic, working as partners and learning from each other. I was also able to work part-time at the Osteopathic Medical School in town, teaching physical assessment to medical students. This helped me expose these students, at an early point in their career, to NPs, who we are, and what we do.

I got married while in Kansas City, and we moved to Maine for her residency. Maine had just recently passed legislation allowing for autonomous practice for NPs, so now what I was considered incompetent and untrained to do in Missouri, I could do in Maine. I took a job at a rural community health center where, by chance, I was employed by a physician I had worked with thirteen years prior in Nome, Alaska! We still work together. She has been there for thirty-five years, and I have been there twenty-two.

I've been working part-time, three days a week, in this practice for twenty-two years, and it's the best job in the world for me.

What has been the most challenging aspect of your career in general?

The most challenging aspect of my career is how the healthcare system focuses on processes, not on patients or outcomes. There is so much measured with computers and checkboxes about what we do, not how we do it, or even more importantly, what the patient wants. It has become an assembly line, a production line, rather than a relationship, a consultation, a sharing of information.

I choose to spend more time with patients, to share information, to give them what they want even if it doesn't match the list of what is supposed to be considered "quality" care.

Do you find the nursing profession stressful? How do you cope with the stress?

I no longer feel this profession is stressful overall. There have been times in my life when I have. There were times, such as working on an air ambulance or in an emergency room, where I thrived on stress.

No, I feel the work is my vocation. I love what I do, and I look forward to going to work each day. I love interacting with people and feel honored and privileged that they share their lives with me. My work gives me life and is deeply rewarding.

For the past twenty-five years, I've been working part time, three days a week, which makes a big difference. I've learned so much from my patients about self-care. Many of the things I do for self-care, eating vegetarian, daily yoga, meditation, and journaling, I also use with my patients. I believe what everyone really wants in life is to feel good and avoid pain. I can help with this. I try to build a relationship of hope with each patient.

How has the COVID-19 pandemic affected your work?

I've learned so much living through this pandemic. In Maine, we prepared but were not hit as hard as other places in the country. I learned about teamwork and flexibility. I also learned that people's needs go on beyond the pandemic. It's stressful for many beyond the pandemic. People need even more time and more focus on their health, beyond the virus. I have made more home visits since the pandemic started and been able to help many elderly or terminally ill people live and even die at home, rather than at an institution where they could have no family around them. My office visits are longer overall since the pandemic.

Have there been times you didn't practice self-care when you knew you needed to?

There were many times, especially early in my career, I was so focused on doing, making a difference, being the best. I pushed myself and worked long and hard hours. I thought money and achievement were such important parts of my life. Now I realize it's all a gift. I recognize that I have nothing to give if I do not take care of myself. My patients have taught me this. In my forty-two years as a nurse, I realize my patients have taught me far more than anyone else ... once I started listening.

What words or ideas would you offer to help nurses in their career that you wish you'd known?

Remember, nursing is about relationship more than process. People need and long for a relationship, someone to listen, to hear them, to advocate for them, to be with them in the challenges and joys of life. There are so many boxes to check and things to click on a computer, but remember to always put connection before content.

Get to know each person before you start doing all the other things. Find out who each person is, who is their support system, how do they cope, what do they enjoy in life. Remember that each person is facing a challenge of fighting a battle that may go well beyond their presenting symptoms. They are longing to share it with someone if we just listen.

What has been the most rewarding aspect of your nursing career?

The patients are certainly the most rewarding aspect of my career. They have taught me so much, given me so much, and helped me grow in so many ways. I love meeting new patients, and I love seeing those I've known for over twenty years. They'll often ask about my family and me or my vacation.

Is there anything else you'd like to share with nurses that could make their lives better?

Work in the system, but you don't have to be *of* the system. Don't be afraid to discover or try new and innovative ways to do things. If we keep doing things the same way all the time, we'll never find new and better ways. This is how discovery and innovation happen. This is how healing happens.

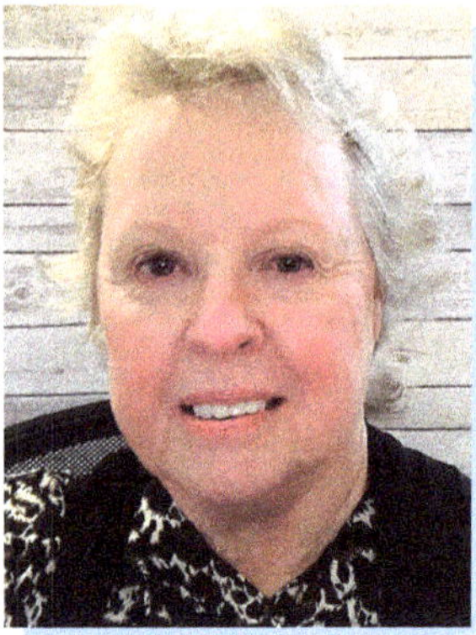 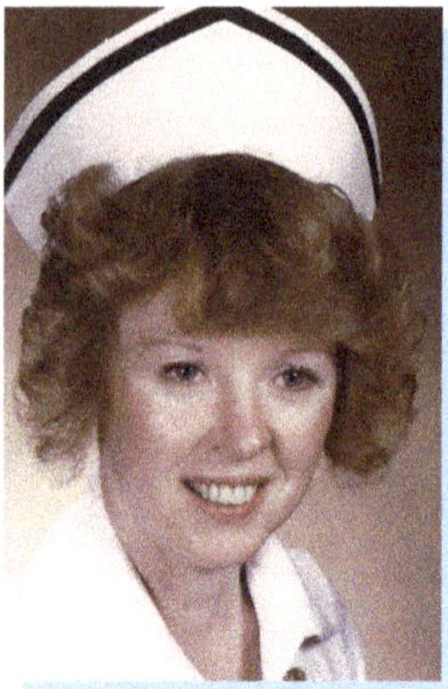

Peggy Mangan, RN

Michigan

What made you decide to become a nurse? Was there someone or an event that influenced you?

What brought me to nursing was that I had a big desire to do something to help others. I was a teenage mom. My husband and I met when I was a junior in high school, and we've been together since I was fourteen. I had a crazy childhood, which was the catalyst for getting out of the house and being eager to get married. I went back to school when my children were young.

I took several aptitude tests to discover which areas I would do best. I'm a helper, so it was either social work or nursing. I went to nursing school in Michigan and became a nurse.

Tell me about your nursing career, such as where you have practiced, what types of facilities you've served in, and how long you have served as a nurse.

When my girls were young, I was a nurse assistant at a doctor's office. Then when they were seven and nine, I graduated from nursing school.

My friend and I went to a job fair held due to a shortage of nurses, and when you walk around, everybody wants you. My friend and I wanted to work in obstetrics, which probably wasn't a good idea. It's not good for a new graduate to go into a high-risk area. But they hired us both, and we went on to work in a high-risk birthing center. It was incredibly intense. But we had our jobs together, and we'd often say to each other, "You take care of me and I'll take care of you."

When a new nurse starts on a unit, she's very often on her own, so if they don't have support, that's the quickest way for them to turn and run; they need the mentoring of a seasoned RN. We went through a twelve-week orientation, which was very helpful; however, that wasn't nearly enough once we got on our own and found out there were so many variations to "normal."

It was a great unit and a great experience. The facility was in Detroit, and I lived north in the suburbs. It was a cultural shock, but I loved the experience. It was very, very challenging for new graduates. I think I was twenty-nine when I graduated after going back to school in my twenties. There were a lot of us older starters who had been moms and then decided to become nurses.

I will never regret it. It was a good choice for me; however, the stress sometimes was just overwhelming.

What has been the most challenging aspect of your career in general?

Starting right out of school was the most challenging aspect for me. They usually like you to get a year in medical/surgical nursing before going to a specialty area, so we had to catch up a lot. But I ended up loving the fast pace. At one point, we delivered 4,000 babies in one year!

I say, "Once a nurse, always a nurse." I've been a nurse for over thirty years. I still have my license, and they're going to take me to the grave with that; it was too difficult to get.

I intended to go into psychiatric nursing, but then I had my OB rotation in school. I thought it was the most amazing experience I'd ever witnessed, aside from my own daughter's birth. But then "new life" didn't end up being the focus.

This was a Level III high-risk birthing facility. We had cardiac moms and diabetic moms. We had moms that had gunshots through the uterus, and we did our own operating. We had four operating rooms and recovery rooms. It encompassed many areas of nursing, including OR, recovery, and special care. What a great experience! It was like an ICU for pregnant ladies with conditions such as pre-eclampsia, cardiac issues, and diabetes.

My saddest memory was of a young woman who died in my arms of an unexpected cranial bleed. I still remember her name, and she's still in my dreams.

Do you find the nursing profession stressful? How do you cope with the stress?

Yes, it was stressful. Any nurse will tell you their job is stressful. You're responsible for people's lives. Each nurse typically only had two rooms, but that means two moms and two babies.

They used to call me the "woo-woo nurse." EFT (Emotional Freedom Techniques) wasn't around then, but I got in on the leading edge of all the alternative and complementary modalities. I practiced self-hypnosis, which was how I got through my exams and my state boards.

I had cancer three times. The first was a melanoma, and it was deep. At the time, there was no chemo for it, only many surgeries. I practiced guided imagery to deal with the cancer. I read Bernie Siegel's book *Love, Medicine and Miracles* religiously over and over. The people that got him into guided imagery were the Simontons, who wrote *Getting Well Again*. They were some of the first to do guided imagery. If I had a bad day, I'd just come home and practice guided imagery.

We didn't always have the luxury of even going somewhere to take a breath, but I used deep breathing simply because it helped. It worked well for stress.

Have there been times you didn't practice self-care when you knew you needed to?

There were times when you just couldn't, because there was no time. You couldn't even go to the bathroom in twelve hours. Nurses all have bladder issues.

When I got hired, twelve-hour shifts were a new concept they were trying out with the new grads. I had to go on nights, which was a difficult shift. I worked an hour away from home. So, it ended up being fourteen-hour days for me. My daughters tell the story that in the mornings, when they'd get up for school, they thought I wasn't home yet. Then they'd look out in the garage and find me sleeping in the car.

What words or ideas would you offer to help nurses in their career that you wish you'd known?

I've done work with some nurses as an EFT practitioner and Matrix Reimprinting, and I strongly recommend them both to help with relieving stress. You can practice EFT discreetly. If I had all this to do again, and I was in one of those emergency surgeries, standing there waiting for the baby to come, I could have practiced EFT on the finger points. Or I could've touched some of the energy points, like the collar bone.

Nurses know what's healthy. They know what's good for them. Self-soothing techniques do help relieve stress.

What has been the most rewarding aspect of your nursing career?

Becoming a good nurse. I was a good nurse and a preceptor to new nurses. Nurses can develop an intuition when it comes to their patients. I always listened to my patients

Is there anything else you'd like to share with nurses that could make their lives better?

Be kind to the new nurses, the "babies," as we referred to them. Be kind to those just coming to the profession. There is an old saying, "Nurses tend to eat their young." There is bullying at times, a pecking order if you will. I was a preceptor on my unit. I had a lot of new "babies."

One instance, after my first cancer, I was scheduled for a routine colonoscopy, but the doctor perforated the wall of my colon. I got peritonitis and was deathly ill. I was packed in ice bags to help lower my dangerously high fever. All through the night, I was slightly aware of this busy person going all around my room doing this and doing that. Finally, when I came around in the morning, she looked at me and said, "You don't remember me, do you?" I replied, "Well, you look familiar." And she said, "I was a student nurse in your unit, and you were the only one nice to me. I took the extra shift to stay with you."

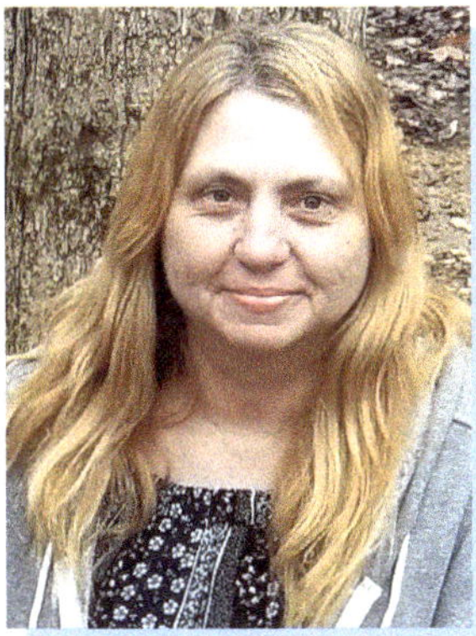

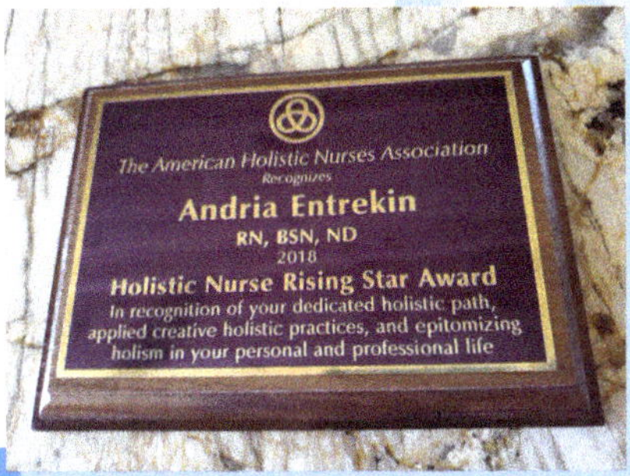
The American Holistic Nurses Association
Recognizes
Andria Entrekin
RN, BSN, ND
2018
Holistic Nurse Rising Star Award
In recognition of your dedicated holistic path, applied creative holistic practices, and epitomizing holism in your personal and professional life

Andria Entrekin, RN, MSN, AHN-BC, HWNC-BC

Mississippi

What made you decide to become a nurse? Was there someone or an event that influenced you?

A gentle push by my parents encouraged me to begin my nursing career as a caring professional.

Tell me about your nursing career, such as where you have practiced, what types of facilities you've served in, and how long you have served as a nurse.

I graduated with my Associate's Degree in Nursing (ADN) in 1990 from Pearl River Community College (PRCC) in Poplarville, Mississippi. In August 2016, I completed my BSN at William Carey University in Hattiesburg, while teaching practical nursing students at PRCC. I completed my MSN from Florida Atlantic University in December 2018. Shortly after completing my MSN, I pursued credentialing as a board-certified advanced holistic nurse and as a health and wellness nurse coach.

I'm presently teaching ADN students at PRCC, and BSN students at the University of Southern Mississippi (USM) in Hattiesburg as a clinical adjunct in the online forum. I have just begun my PhD with William Carey University as of June this year.

I have worked in many clinical settings (orthopedics, oncology, outpatient surgery, extended care, etc.) over the years as a travel nurse, staff nurse, and clinical instructor. I'm now seeking employment chiefly online as a move away from the clinical setting and to provide more flexibility with home and family life.

What has been the most challenging aspect of your career in general?

The most challenging, somewhat discouraging, aspect of my career is the inability to find full-time employment within my specialty as a holistic nurse. I truly desire to teach at an endorsed school by the American Holistic Nurses Credentialing Corporation (AHNCC) or at least be able to teach a holistic elective or a course with a holistic focus (such as holistic nursing assessment). A huge obstacle seems to be the biomedical model of providing care interweaved in nursing curriculums. I am hoping, with the collaboration of many others, to place holistic nursing on the map in the nursing curriculum within my home state (Mississippi) during the pursuit of my PhD in Nursing Education and Administration.

Do you find the nursing profession stressful? How do you cope with the stress?

The nursing profession has always been stressful. I feel, in general, that I cope very well with stress, but much of my coping has been improved by professional experience and maturity. I wish that I'd been introduced to holistic nursing concepts (self-care, self-reflection, self-awareness) along with the entire holistic nursing mindset at the beginning of my nursing career as an associate degree nurse. Furthermore, I've conducted surveys and held holistic chapter meetings (focusing on self-care) among associate degree faculty and students to offer such an elective in holistic nursing. Still, without funding and/or future publication, their interest may be as if it were nonexistent.

How has the COVID-19 pandemic affected your work?

I've been minimally affected by the pandemic associated with the COVID-19 virus. In fact, my life has included more of what I've wanted in my career (to teach online, be home more with family).

Have there been times you didn't practice self-care when you knew you needed to?

There have been times that I have not practiced self-care in attempting to keep up with my many responsibilities as a wife, mother, grandmother, student, nurse, etc. However, I attempt every day to practice what I preach. Before the virus (outbreak, fear, economic meltdown, social distancing), I was planning a regional self-care conference with Terri Roberts, executive director of the American Holistic Nurses Association (AHNA), to be held in September of this year. It now seems that even this very needed event will be postponed due to the COVID-19 pandemic.

What words or ideas would you offer to help nurses in their career that you wish you'd known?

I suggest that the basic concepts of holistic nursing, including the Five Core Values of Holistic Nursing, be taught as the foundation for all nurses at the undergraduate or community college level within their program of study in all schools of nursing. To ever achieve healing in healthcare, healing in professionals, and healing in clients, healing must begin within each of us. I feel that nursing professionals and students agree on this concept, but the implementation and interweaving of holistic-nursing concepts in our schools of nursing are what is needed.

What has been the most rewarding aspect of your nursing career?

The most rewarding aspect of my nursing career has been the pursuit and completion of my MSN degree with Florida Atlantic University (FAU). FAU's school of nursing is endorsed by the American Holistic Nurses Credentialing Center (AHNCC) and offers a nursing curriculum of holistic nursing courses.

Is there anything else you'd like to share with nurses that could make their lives better?

I wrote a poem for an assignment while attending FAU and it's included in this book. Although the poem is addressed to holistic nurses, I feel the message is important for all nurses everywhere. I hope you enjoy it.

Thinking Mind, Compassion Heart

By Andria Entrekin RN, MSN, AHN-BC, HWNC-BC

Dedicated to Holistic Nurses Everywhere

Today I am aware of who I am.

My beliefs, values, feelings.

Today I am aware of my sensations,
perceptions, and judgments.

My need to cry, pray, forgive, forget, laugh, and love.

Today I look in the mirror.

My reflection of who I am.
I am becoming more authentic and mindful.

Today I value myself for who I am.

My resources help me heal. I am integrating
self-awareness, self-care, self-healing,
and self-responsibility. I am reaching for the stars!
My goal is my highest healing potential!

Today I honor my complete self.

My psychological, social, cultural, intellectual,
and spiritual self, if I allow it, guides me by bringing
attention to those needs that only I know about.

Today I am healing.

My ways of healing are facilitated by
self-reflection and self-care.
I am developing a deep self-reflection.
I accept that healing is a lifelong process and that
we each heal by different means.

Today I am seeking harmony.

My silencing of noise, my observance of nature,
my moments in prayer, my acceptance of life
as it unfolds, and my healing journey brings harmony.

Today I practice centering.

My mind still is wrapping itself around centering.
I am practicing this. I have learned how to become
calm in stressful situations.

Today I am making plans for the future.

My future involves caring for others
through education and implementation
of caring-healing relationships
in all that I do.

Today I am aware of who I am.

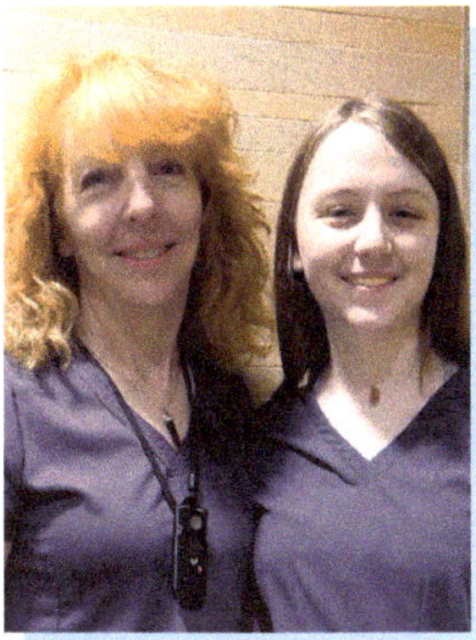

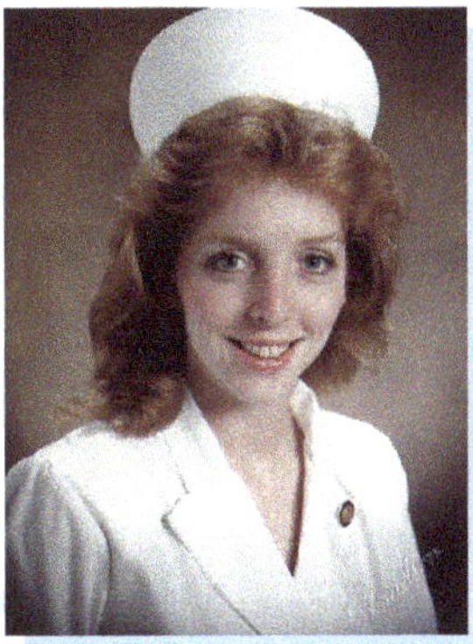

Nancy Beck, BSN, RN

Missouri

What made you decide to become a nurse? Was there someone or an event that influenced you?

I always knew I was going to be a nurse. Santa brought me a nurse's bag when I was in the second grade and I used to pass out Red Hot candies as "medicine." When I was a teenager, my grandfather died unexpectantly from a heart attack, and my grandmother died of breast cancer. I wanted to be that nurse who I hope they had taking care of them.

Tell me about your nursing career, such as where you have practiced, what types of facilities you've served in, and how long you have served as a nurse.

I have been working as a cardiac nurse for thirty-three years. My hospital has received recognition for its cardiac care, and our program has the top recognition for cardiovascular surgeons. We've also received Magnet designation three times.

What has been the most challenging aspect of your career in general?

The most challenging thing in nursing is the moment when I need to be in multiple places at once to assist multiple patients, and I can only be in one place at a time.

Do you find the nursing profession stressful? How do you cope with the stress?

Nursing can be very stressful. It's through my spiritual growth that I've been able to handle being a nurse—finding that place within myself to witness a person's unfolding, rather than to judge it. It makes it easier to be supportive of patients and their families.

How has the COVID-19 pandemic affected your work?

Learning to live with the situation of COVID-19 in day-to-day life has been a significant challenge. Watching it all unfold and knowing within myself what is going to happen next. Little bits and pieces of information come from different sources. It's very concerning how all of this is happening.

Have there been times you didn't practice self-care when you knew you needed to?

I am fairly consistent. I try to rest when I need to. I stay off the internet and computers when too much information is coming at once. I eat a little too much candy, but it doesn't affect my weight.

What words or ideas would you offer to help nurses in their career that you wish you'd known?

My daughter is in nursing school. I didn't encourage or discourage her from being a nurse. She has watched me and knows what's needed, as far as holidays away from the family and long shifts. There were a couple of points I wanted to make to her. One is that you really have to be passionate about being a nurse. If you're not, your life will be very unhappy. It's a hard job. The other is that there are so many options. If you start in one area and don't like it, there are other areas of specialty, from the bedside, teaching, computers, or working as a medical rep.

What has been the most rewarding aspect of your nursing career?

Going to work every day with the expectation that I'll be giving excellent patient care. This month I walked into a room and introduced myself like I have done so many times. The patient looked at me and said, "I remember you. You are my angel. You may not remember this, but three years ago, I was here and had lung surgery to remove cancer. You walked into the room and could see I was in rough shape. Before you walked out of the room, you made a commitment to me that you were going to get me taken care of. You apologized for the prior nurse and explained that normally she wouldn't have allowed this to happen. You then got my pain under control. I'll never forget you." A couple of days later, the patient was walking in the halls with her husband, and she stopped to introduce the two of us. She turned to her husband and said, "Do you remember the angel I had told you about? Here she is." They went on to discuss the many conversations that they had over what had been a trauma prior to my care and how important I had been to her.

Is there anything else you'd like to share with nurses that could make their lives better?

Take care of yourself. Learn to say "No" when you don't want to work that extra shift. For the first five years of my career, I always said: "Yes." I started to resent my work. I also discovered we always needed help yet they weren't hiring new staff. The need never stopped. I became much happier when I learned to say "No."

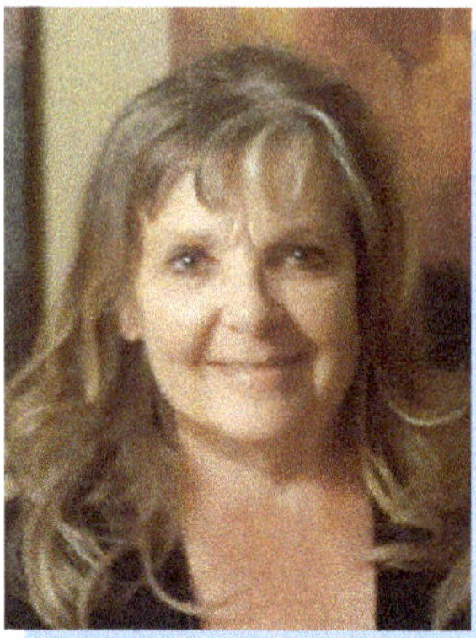

Debera Charlton, MSN, RN

Montana

What made you decide to become a nurse? Was there someone or an event that influenced you?

I was very privileged to meet Inez, a caregiver, when I was seven years old. Inez was taking care of an elderly woman who was comatose and actively dying. Inez brought the breadth of humanity in her care with compassion and dignity. Family members never seemed to go into the room to interact with this woman, but Inez consistently engaged and spoke to her as if this woman was still awake and participating in life. She groomed her daily and invited me in to help. I learned to braid hair while helping with her "activities of daily living" (ADLs).

Inez would also sing and play the violin to this woman and let her know what was going on throughout the day. I knew from this experience, as a seven-year-old, that I wanted to make a difference and follow in those footsteps to care for others in a way that made a difference!

Tell me about your nursing career, such as where you have practiced, what types of facilities you've served in, and how long you have served as a nurse.

I've been a nurse for twenty-one years! It was a long road from age seven to the day I got my degree for sure. I was a stay-at-home mom and went back to school at age thirty-six. I was much older than the average student, but it is never too late.

I have been privileged to work in both the private and public sectors of healthcare. I have worked on the medical/surgical floor all shifts, on OB as both staff and as a director of a women and children's unit, as a quality management specialist, ambulatory care nurse manager, designated learning officer for a government-based hospital, and as an adjunct professor for nursing for both a community college and a private university. I have also been a formal preceptor for students and new staff throughout my entire nursing career in any position I served.

What has been the most challenging aspect of your career in general?

The most challenging aspect of my career has been working in unhealthy, toxic work environments where leadership does not value, hear, or acknowledge the voice of the front-line nursing staff. Learning techniques of not giving up and continuing to speak up, negotiating a win-win better way, always keeping the heart of my motivation in check, and genuine connectedness has helped temper these challenges.

Another challenge has been not having the opportunity to debrief and take time to recover when difficult patient-care situations came up.

Other challenges include finding a way to move forward when personal values no longer align with corporate and facility values, plus knowing when to leave or move on with courage and grace.

Do you find the nursing profession stressful? How do you cope with the stress?

Of course, but not all stress is bad. Stress can motivate, create resilience, create change, regroup one to focus and re-evaluate, and challenge one. Stress can build self-efficacy and autonomy.

I cope with stress through meditation and relaxation techniques, journaling, concentrating on my resources, reminding myself of and developing my strengths, practicing optimism, being aware of and refocusing my perceptions and seeing the potential benefit of the current situation I'm facing, incorporating the practice of my daily gratitude jar, spending meaningful time with close friends and family, and removing myself from toxic relationships and situations.

How has the COVID-19 pandemic affected your work?

Yes, COVID-19 has affected my work in many ways: reorienting to floor nursing to be ready to cover staff during a potential COVID-19 surge, sending staff to cover other facilities that are in a surge (this was very distressing at times knowing they were in high-risk work, and I could only send my support and not be with them), creating levity when needed, embracing and working through grief as it comes, learning to work from home with virtual modalities, learning new techniques for leading teams, connecting with families in new ways other than face-to-face, integrating and implementing new care practices for staff, assuring constant communication with ever-changing practice and PPE directives, and maintaining self-healthy practices as well as for family and colleagues.

Have there been times you didn't practice self-care when you knew you needed to?

Indeed. These included times of working sixteen-eighteen hour shifts to cover patient care when staff called off, saying "Yes" when I should have said "No," skipping meals and breaks on shift after shift, canceling vacations to assure the work got done, tolerating both unhealthy and toxic working environments and leadership, not speaking up when I should have, speaking up ineffectively and inappropriately, not working through grief, not debriefing enough when difficult patient situations occurred, and the well-known self-care elements of lack of sleep, exercise, and healthy eating.

What words or ideas would you offer to help nurses in their career that you wish you'd known?

Create your legacy early on in your career. What do you want to be remembered for after each shift, each patient interaction, each day, each week, and each year?

Create a personal mission statement that aligns with your values for nursing, self, and family. Review and update each annually.

I was so blessed to have a patient help me write my legacy early in my career, from the patient's point of view, which helped me align my values of how to make a difference in patient care every day. We wrote together in a treasured journal over a six-week period when I was taking care of this patient.

I also encourage all to create a personal and professional development plan annually for the next six months, next year, and next five years with SMART goals (*see* Glossary) to develop continued growth. Create a "toolbelt" of strong communication tools for how to have successful difficult conversations, negotiate, create connectedness, build strong interprofessional relationships, focus on and develop your strengths rather than your weaknesses, speak up, and partner with the patient with a "whole health" approach to care.

And, never forfeit your priorities.

What has been the most rewarding aspect of your nursing career?

The most rewarding aspect of my career is that I have been honored to care for the entire circle of life, from "catching" those newborns taking their first breath, to holding the hand of those taking their last breath. The similarities and stark differences on both sides of life has broadened my life views, enhanced my tolerance and appreciation for diversity, provided me with the ability to wholly embrace miracles, cultivate greater compassion, provide meaningful, tailored nursing care that supports variation to meet the individual's needs, and develop positive interprofessional relationships because it now takes multiple disciplines working together to take care of the patient. It is a team approach with the patient at the center.

Is there anything else you'd like to share with nurses that could make their lives better?

Remember your worth, focus on your strengths, share your knowledge, and embrace the circle of care, which is to take care of yourself, take care of others, and take care of the place/unit/culture you work in.

Continue to learn and grow professionally and personally. Find a good formal mentor, develop strong communication skills that always start with motivation from your heart, take care of you, embrace the positive side of stress, reflect daily, integrate daily practices that enhance self-care, regularly set goals and create a solid written journey of how you will get there. Remember your legacy and look ahead at how you can make a difference in someone's life every day.

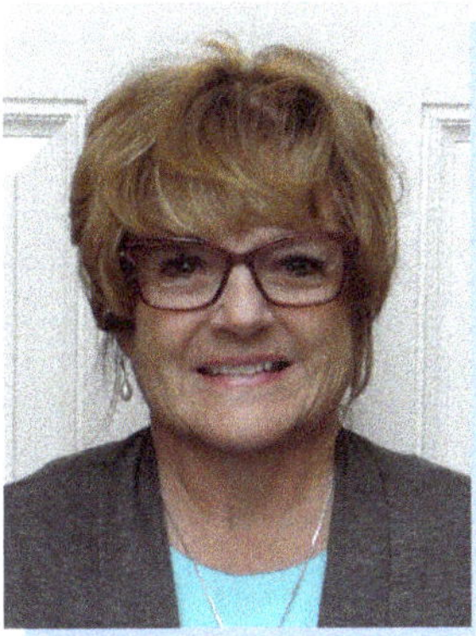 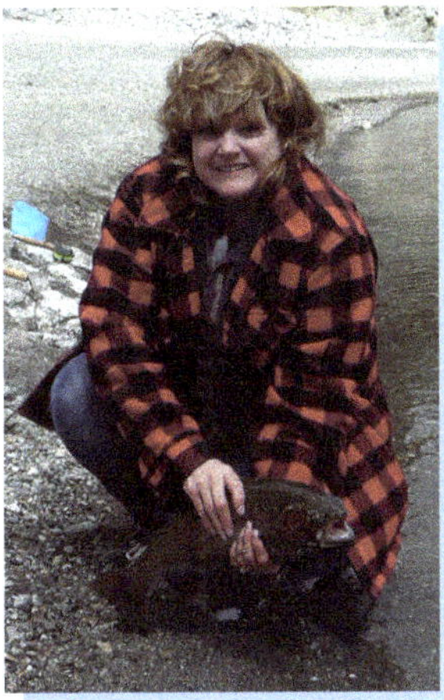

Jerri Kettman, RNC

Montana

What made you decide to become a nurse? Was there someone or an event that influenced you?

I think I've always been a caregiver and have had that "caregiver's spirit" in me.

In my senior year, there was a class I had to take, and I started volunteering at the residential home and school for special needs children and adults. That led to a position with special education, and I was there for about seven years. Then I met my husband and got married. We traveled for a few months and settled in Montana because we love the mountains and the outdoors. When we got there, it seemed like the nursing theme kept coming up. This was back in 1981, and there was a shortage of nurses in Montana.

My father-in-law's health was declining, so we headed back to the Midwest to help take care of him. And the nurse theme continued to come up there, too. I had the thought that maybe this is where I need to focus. I had a couple of aunts who were nurses, and my sister is a nurse, and she persuaded me to look at nursing, suggesting that it might be a good fit for me. I started out by earning my LPN diploma, and then I wanted to test the waters to see if nursing really was for me. And I loved it! I was hooked. I love patient care, and I love teaching. I worked as an LPN while continuing to get my RN degree. So that's how I got into the nursing profession.

Tell me about your nursing career, such as where you have practiced, what types of facilities you've served in, and how long you have served as a nurse.

Well, I'm one of those "seasoned nurses" with thirty-eight years of experience. I used to say "old nurse," but I like the term "seasoned nurse" better. As an LPN, I worked at an extended care facility. It was a private facility, an extended care step down from hospital care, which was my first real experience with team care. I was the LPN and had three nursing aides working with me.

Then I got my RN degree, and there was a position in the community available. They were looking for a school nurse for developmentally disabled adults. With my background in special education, it was a good fit and I did that for about a year.

We set a goal to head back to Montana, and that's when I took a full-time job at the community hospital on the medical floor, working night shift. It was a great experience, and I had great nurse mentors. I worked there for twenty-three years.

Then they started talking about opening up an acute psychiatric unit. I accepted the opportunity to work there with a great team of nurses, psychiatrists, social workers, and psychologists. We developed policies, procedures, treatment plans, and various therapy modalities. I worked there for eighteen years.

And then, another adventure started; I worked with hospice for five years as a case manager. It was an interesting experience when I first started because I'd been on one end of the spectrum, helping suicidal people want to live, and then in hospice, I was working on the other end of the spectrum, the end of life. It was an interesting time. My psychiatry nursing had prepared me and helped me realize it was a good balance for me.

While I was working with hospice, I worked with a lot of veterans, allowing me to be connected with the VA hospital and the nurses there.

As I came closer to the end of my nursing career, I thought maybe I needed to go back to psych nursing, which I love doing.

I got a call from the chief of the psych department at the VA for an interview, and I was hired as a crisis triage PTSD nurse. I had all these titles, and I was not really sure what I was going to be doing, but I was up for a new adventure. And it was a great experience. I did that for about two or three years, before becoming a nurse manager for nine years. I supervised RNs, LPNs, medical support assistance, social workers, psychologists, and nurse practitioners.

I'm an RN, a nurse, not a subject expert in social work or psychology. I even supervised a couple of psychiatrists. It was a great experience and I loved it. I loved my team, and it was a great opportunity. But then I had a nurse that was transferring to another VA, and I had been missing patient care, so I asked my supervisor if I could be reassigned to this case manager position. It's clinical care, and I get to spend time every day with veterans and manage their patient care. That's what I'm doing right now, and I love it.

What has been the most challenging aspect of your career in general?

When I first started, the biggest challenge for me was balancing my family and work. As a nurse, you're working every other weekend and working holidays, but you need to be able to find a balance. I have a great family and a lot of good support from a great network of nurses. Whenever I had a challenge, it always seemed like I had support there to help me work through it, so I was fortunate that way.

I've seen a shift over the years with the next generation coming into nursing. I think they're more prepared for self-care than I ever was in my training. We didn't have that training. We were focused on clinical skills, medical/surgical, and pharmacy, but nothing about self-care back then. So it's an exciting time for nurses. I think there's been a good shift.

Do you find the nursing profession stressful? How do you cope with the stress?

Nursing can be stressful. You're multitasking, triaging, and working with multiple disciplines. There are the dynamics of the patient and the family. It can be stressful, but I've been fortunate over the years because I've worked with psychiatrists, medical doctors, psychologists, social workers, and RNs. And I've had time to debrief and to process, which has helped me cope with my stress. When I've had a challenging day, I try to look at what went well and what areas I could improve. And I get feedback from my mentors and my peers. I'm always looking for ways to improve. I also read leadership books and self-help books.

I tried to set an example for my peers and my nursing and clinical staff. It seems like it's easy for us to look at the negative, but I always try to bring up what went well, and I tried to bring that out to them.

I love rocks. I have rocks all over my desk, and I give rocks to different patients and nurses. I have this gratitude rock, and I've shared that many times to different people when they're in need.

Have there been times you didn't practice self-care when you knew you needed to?

At the beginning of my career, there were times I felt overwhelmed. I know as a new nurse, your first death, your first trauma, or first emergency situation can be overwhelming. But as a psychiatric nurse, we teach and promote self-care, and we teach recovery. So, I tried to walk the walk with myself and provide some guidance.

That said, I think nurses have a great network of friends, peers, coworkers, and mentors. And they don't hold back. They'll call me on it and say, "It looks like you're not taking care of yourself. You need to take some time." So I've been fortunate with that. And I have another mentor who knows I'll call her on it too. We have this pact to be there for each other.

What words or ideas would you offer to help nurses in their career that you wish you'd known?

It's hard work to be a nurse. You really need to pay attention to how you're feeling. More awareness is needed to avoid fatigue and burnout.

It's important for nurses to be in tune with themselves and to recognize when they need to take some time off or take a break to go for a hike or fly fishing or spend time with creative hobbies, like quilting, knitting, or painting.

Sometimes we advise nurses to take a break from nursing. My generation always felt guilty when we called in sick, or when we took time off, because we felt that was a burden to our coworkers having to pick up our patient load. But I think it's shifting because the new, younger nurses are starting with a more solid idea of work-life balance. They work hard, but they also take time off with less guilt. When I lecture at the college about self-care, these young nurses are already in tune with it.

What has been the most rewarding aspect of your nursing career?

I've learned over the years, as I witnessed it or experienced it myself, that the little things you do or say can make a big difference in someone's life. And that's especially rewarding when it comes back to you.

Through reflection, I realize I found my purpose when I was doing hospice. I really connected with that. I was always amazed at how open the patient and the families were, letting a stranger come into their house in the most emotional, intimate time of their life.

I could write a book about the amazing experiences I've had. While working in hospice, I had the privilege to be a nurse for a couple of patients with mental health challenges and I took care of them when they came into the acute psychiatric unit.

There was one patient that I was a little concerned about, wondering how he would respond to me being his hospice nurse. He recognized me and asked if I was going to be his nurse and I thought,

"Oh, I don't know how this is going to go." So I said, "Only if you will allow me to be your nurse." And then he proceeded to talk with me about a time maybe thirty years before. He remembered how kind and respectful I was toward him and he'd never forgotten that. It was extremely touching.

There are so many opportunities in nursing, and I've been truly fortunate. I think the sky's the limit, and it's been a great ride.

I've been volunteering at the community hospital with a program called No One Dies Alone (NODA). Because of my work with hospice, I'm comfortable with end of life. There's about twenty-five or thirty of us that volunteer to sit with patients so that they don't pass on alone; there's always someone with them. It's a great program, and it has been a wonderful experience.

Is there anything else you'd like to share with nurses that could make their lives better?

No, I think this covers it. This opportunity has been a really positive experience, and I had to pause and reflect on your questions. One night, I woke up about three o'clock in the morning and thought, "Oh, yeah, I forgot about that." It's been fun reflecting on my career as a nurse. I wouldn't change a thing.

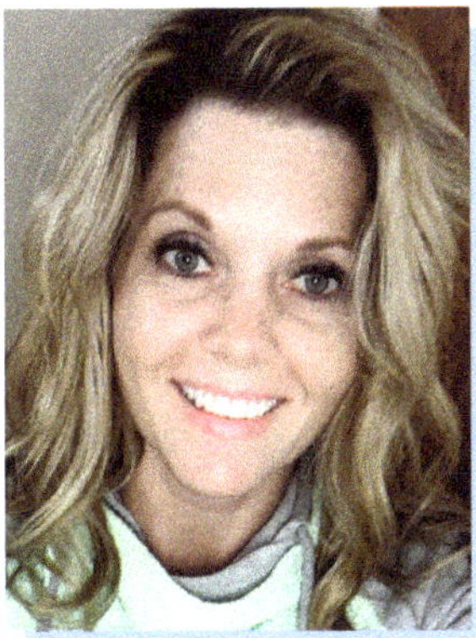

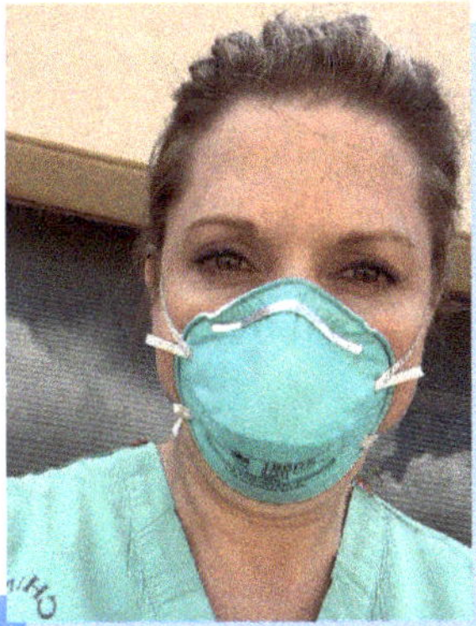

Katie Temple, MN, RN, CNL

Montana

What made you decide to become a nurse? Was there someone or an event that influenced you?

When I was pregnant with my first child, the nurse practitioner who worked with my doctor was amazing and inspired me to start looking into a nursing career.

Tell me about your nursing career, such as where you have practiced, what types of facilities you've served in, and how long you have served as a nurse.

I've been a nurse for fourteen years, and it's been an honor to give back to our veterans at the VA hospital for all those years. I worked as an inpatient nurse for a couple of years and then moved to primary care for thirteen years, and now I'm working in education.

What has been the most challenging aspect of your career in general?

The most challenging aspect of my career has been advancing my education while working as a nurse. When you have a family and need to work, but yet want to continue your education and self-growth, at certain points in the education process, it can be challenging to manage all those pieces.

Do you find the nursing profession stressful? How do you cope with the stress?

For me, the nursing profession is not extremely stressful. I love it so much that I take it as a positive challenge. I will say working in certain areas is definitely more stressful than others, but I find that a positive outlook, working as a team, and my faith are what get me through the stress.

How has the COVID-19 pandemic affected your work?

I had the opportunity to volunteer and be deployed to help in a COVID-19 hotspot on the Navajo Nation. I've never done anything like this before and felt if there was somewhere in need, then I should go and be of service.

I went and helped for two weeks on an all-COVID-19 unit in a small, rural hospital. This experience was very emotional, stressful, trying, exhausting, but yet rewarding and fulfilling at the same time.

COVID-19 patients cannot have visitors. They are all by themselves, so the only human interaction they get is with the healthcare workers. I realized my purpose was to be there to help with medical care, but in addition to that, showing compassion and empathy to another human going through something difficult all by themselves. Many of the people didn't leave the hospital or make it, and many were intubated and flown out. I did witness three who improved enough to return home, and it was so exciting that we lined the halls and cheered for them as that outcome wasn't typical with this illness.

Montana has been lucky not to be one of the hotspots with COVID-19, therefore going somewhere else that was struggling to fight this illness opened my eyes to the severity and how it is affecting people right here close to home. It's so easy to forget and not notice the impact of certain issues when they're not impacting your everyday life. When

I came back from helping with COVID-19, I had to be quarantined because I'd been dipped in the COVID-19 bucket. Luckily, I came out clean and healthy, and I'm very thankful and blessed for that as so many people aren't.

When I returned from my two weeks away, and time in quarantine, I had time to reflect on the experience. It showed me how every day is a blessing, every person deserves compassion, and every human has a story. We can all impact each other positively if we take the time to see each other and listen to each other's stories. I definitely appreciate the blessings I have daily. COVID-19 and that experience helped me to cherish the things in life that matter, because one minute you can be fine and the next you never know.

Have there been times you didn't practice self-care when you knew you needed to?

Being a nurse, I always put the focus on helping others versus helping myself. I recently had major surgery and needed to focus on myself and ask others for help in ways I never have before. That was very difficult for me, but yet I learned a great lesson: it's okay to ask for help and spend time on yourself for your own physical, mental, and spiritual well-being. By doing this, I could be better for all those around me whom I wanted to care for in my personal and professional life.

What words or ideas would you offer to help nurses in their career that you wish you'd known?

Find a mentor early in your career, somebody you trust and look up to. They can help be a guide for you and your career, see strengths in you that you may not see, help push you when you don't want to move, help hold you accountable for goals and dreams you have voiced, and help you to see opportunities you would've maybe never seen for yourself. I was not looking for a mentor but was blessed in getting one early on in my nursing career, and she has helped me immensely see things within myself and potential I didn't see.

What has been the most rewarding aspect of your nursing career?

The most rewarding aspect of my nursing career has been working with veterans. Being able to give back to those who have served our country has been more than I could've asked for.

Is there anything else you'd like to share with nurses that could make their lives better?

Take every opportunity you can to help yourself grow personally and professionally, even if it seems scary. Many times, you must push through the fear to see your amazing purpose and potential on the other side. Support those around you, as we all have different strengths, and if we work together, we can reach amazing outcomes.

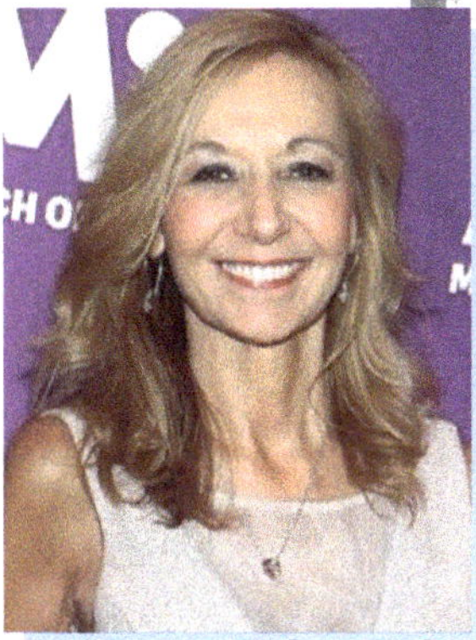

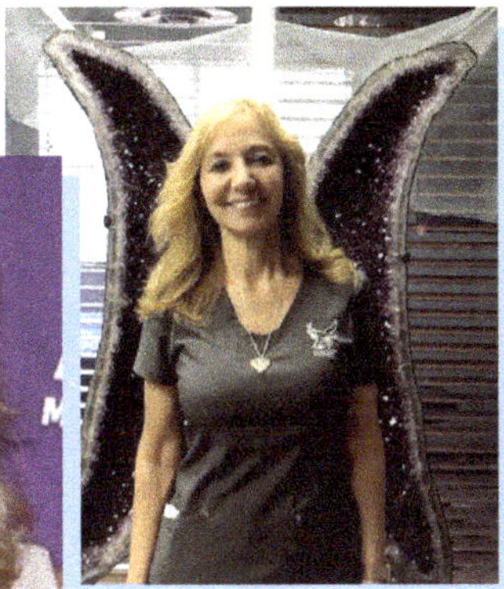

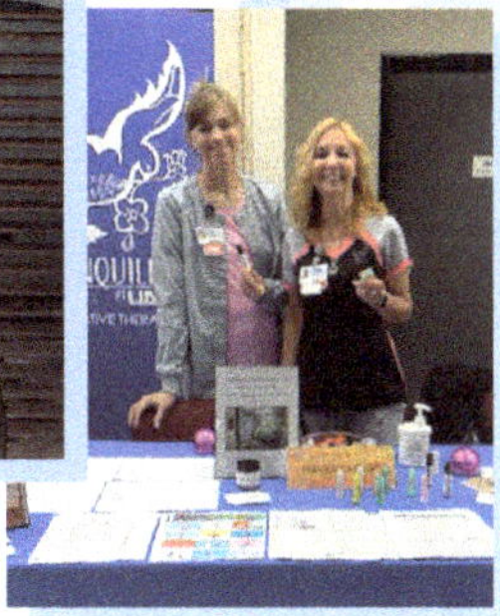

Michelle McGrorey, BSN, RN, OCN, HTCP, NCCA, HMIP, HBN-BC

Nevada

What made you decide to become a nurse? Was there someone or an event that influenced you?

I was sixteen years old and saw my grandmother die of metastatic breast cancer. I had wanted to be a physician since I was seven years old, but this event changed my mind. I watched the doctors and nurses take care of my grandmother, and the nurses were the ones showing compassion and care to her and my family. They inspired me to go into nursing.

Their caring attitude, compassion to push for more pain meds to keep her comfortable, and the way the nurses cared for her while she was dying is forever etched in my brain. Just rolling her in the bed would fracture her ribs from the metastasis. The nurses would include us in her care and not make us feel left out. The doctors avoided talking about her imminent death.

Even at sixteen years of age, I knew she was dying. The nurses acknowledged her condition to us and were realistic. The doctors would come in the room and avoid eye contact. The nurses would look me in the eyes, and at times have tears in their own eyes as they rallied for more pain control for her. I knew I wanted to be a nurse after this.

This career path would enable me to be at the forefront and care for people when they were most vulnerable, to be an advocate for the patient, and to support the family. So, at the age of sixteen, I decided nursing was my path. That was thirty-eight years ago. I never regretted it.

Tell me about your nursing career, such as where you have practiced, what types of facilities you've served in, and how long you have served as a nurse.

I've been a nurse for over thirty-eight years. I have worked in almost every area of nursing from medical/surgical, pediatrics, labor and delivery, home health, public health, emergency department (ED), education, management, oncology, and integrative therapies. I've worked in big cities and rural areas.

I started out in New York in a county hospital for ten years and then married a family practice physician and moved to rural areas in New York, Nevada, and Texas. This really opened my eyes as rural nursing is very different from nursing in a large hospital with support all around you. In my rural nursing days, I may be running a small ED, working with trauma victims, strokes, etc., and mixing our own drugs because we didn't have a pharmacist in-house. It was a crazy world "in the field," but it was a great experience. I also managed a rural clinic while in the small town of Hawthorne, Nevada.

I worked in rural nursing for thirteen years. Then I moved to Las Vegas and worked in oncology. That was the *last* department I wanted to work in; I had asked God to put me anywhere but oncology! So, of course, I landed in oncology in a large county hospital in Las Vegas. I expected to stay six months and transfer out. Fast forward to thirteen years later, I was still working in oncology. I loved it!

In 2010, during my sixth year in oncology, I took a Healing Touch class, and it changed my life. I became very involved with holistic nursing and started doing Healing Touch on my oncology patients. Then I started using aromatherapy with them—all with my manager's approval. I was working thirty-six hours on the oncology floor as a staff nurse, and I would come in for four hours each week and work with oncology patients doing holistic modalities. I continued doing this and then started including staff as well as patients.

We had an administrative change and received a new CNO in 2016. I asked for her approval to continue providing these services to patients and staff. When she found out what my colleague and I were doing, she asked us to start an entirely new department in the hospital using integrative modalities. It was three years ago that Tranquility at University Medical Center in Las Vegas, Nevada, was born!

What started out as a few hours per week back in 2010 has blossomed to a full-time, hospital-wide practice. This is completely nurse-driven, and we see as many staff as we do patients. We go to the bedside and educate on integrative therapies and provide services such as Healing Touch, music, breath work, guided imagery, and aromatherapy. We teach patients, staff, and the community on these evidence-based modalities. It has been an incredible few years!

What has been the most challenging aspect of your career in general?

There have been many challenging areas of my nursing career, and I've seen many changes over the years. At first, in the 1980s, the challenges were mainly between the nurses and physicians. Finding the road between following their orders and questioning their orders was something you didn't do. My first day on the job, my charge nurse had me carrying the ashtray around for the Medical Director to catch his ashes as he rounded!

Times have certainly changed! This went on for years, and then nurses were seen as more influential in patient care. We got a voice.

We became advocates for our patients and weren't afraid to question the doctors and be more involved with educating our patients.

I remember back in the 1980s, you couldn't even tell the patient their blood pressure. The doctor had to tell them. We were limited on what we could say or teach the patients. The focus was also on treatment, not health or prevention.

There were also definitely challenges with the changes in nursing, as far as the delivery of care. I started with very hands-on care, providing back rubs, etc., what I call Florence Nightingale nursing: very involved with the whole patient, the family, and the environment.

There was a massive shift with the addition of computers to a hands-off type of care. I found that very disturbing. That is one of the reasons I enjoy integrative therapies and holistic nursing so much; it brings us back to the basics with the addition of wonderful tools to help patients and staff.

We have also had the challenges from the swing to pain as the fifth vital sign, to the profession being afraid to provide pain control; it's a complete pendulum swing. Pain control is a difficult thing in this day and age. It's a balancing act of providing suitable pain medication, along with holistic modalities, to help put the patient in the best possible position to heal. There has been a large shift from just treating the symptoms for patients to also focusing on health, prevention, and stress management.

There have been so many challenges along this journey! When I started providing integrative therapies to staff and patients, my colleagues and the physicians thought I was crazy. My own family thought I was crazy. I was only providing science-based modalities, but it caused a lot of stress with my relationships. I was always very well-respected as a nurse, and all of a sudden, I was doing energy work on patients! So many people thought I was crazy. It actually contributed to my divorce.

But I knew the importance of teaching patients and staff about stress reduction years ago. I kept moving forward. During this time since 2010, I obtained my Healing Touch certification, became a certified aromatherapist, then a National Association for Holistic Aromatherapy (NAHA) Clinical Aromatherapist, and a HeartMath Interventions Provider. I was also certified in oncology nursing. Now I get consults to see patients as other providers do.

The physicians and nurses can put an order in the computer, and we go see patients. We have grown in our hospital from nobody knowing who we were or what we did, to working with every department, with the patients and staff. We also hold classes to teach staff and the community holistic modalities to help them mitigate symptoms, stay healthy, reduce stress, and learn different tools to help them.

Do you find the nursing profession stressful? How do you cope with the stress?

Including all the above, I do find the nursing profession can be very stressful. There's also a lot of stress from incivility and bullying. It seems to be in every department of nursing from the top down. I feel that as nurses, we have many stressors. Stress to provide the best care to patients and include their families, to continue the never-ending journey of becoming the best nurse by staying educated and always learning, including being technologically savvy. We must juggle the computer era with hands-on nursing. We must continue to balance work and family. We are the most trusted profession, but the least healthy.

We must learn to focus on self-care. Learning to care for ourselves is not selfish. Self-care is a necessity. We cannot take care of others without putting ourselves in the best mode we can be in. To do that, we must learn to take time to do self-care, learn tools to use to de-stress, to become patient and staff advocates, to get involved in our work environment by joining councils and having a voice.

I cope with stress by practicing what I preach. I focus on the three main pillars: food, exercise, and sleep. I also incorporate meditation, yoga, essential oils, biofeedback, breath work, and other science-based modalities to help keep me focused and de-stressed. I read the Bible as it keeps me balanced for my spirituality. I love going outside and "earthing," I journal, etc. I use many different tools to keep me in the best mode I can put myself in.

How has the COVID-19 pandemic affected your work?

COVID-19 has affected everyone. Our new normal is a totally new way of thinking and being. It has people living in fear. We have seen loved ones die, coworkers get ill, and continue to live in fear that we or our loved ones will get sick. There have been no in-person meetings; everything has gone to virtual. It has brought out the best in some people and the worst in others. We are all still navigating this new world.

We have seen or been involved with people dying alone. People unable to identify their loved ones or get their bodies back home due to COVID. People have lost their jobs due to the economics of all of this. The world is turned upside down. Since I go throughout the hospital, providing support to patients and staff, I have heard so many stories, gut-wrenching stories. I feel like we're all in the war zone.

Non-COVID patients are affected by this also. The trauma patients, the labor and delivery patients ... This has touched everything and everyone. I find by the end of the workweek, even with trying to use all the tools in my toolbox, I am emotionally, mentally, and physically exhausted. I need to recharge every week. It has taken a toll on us.

I was getting a little depressed for a while. I'm very social, and this caused me to halt all social activities. On a good note, I've learned to love to be home and focus on different things. It has brought my family, which was already close, even closer. I have learned to FaceTime with my significant other when I'm quarantining myself from exposure to COVID-19.

Have there been times you didn't practice self-care when you knew you needed to?

There are times I knew I should do my self-care but didn't. I've been making sure I take time for the self-care, because if I don't, my health and my work suffers. I can't give to the patients if I'm depleted. I have incorporated a brisk walk outside for one of my breaks during the day. I get outside in the fresh air and walk around the hospital building. That fifteen minutes is priceless, and I feel refreshed and renewed. I take advantage of the Tranquility rooms I opened throughout the hospital. We can go into a Tranquility room for fifteen minutes and use oils, the Care Channel, and renew. We have books in the rooms, breathing exercises, yoga mats, rain sticks, etc.

I have found when I let myself get depleted, my mood is not as positive as it should be. I am not as focused. I have a hard time centering and being present.

The importance of self-care cannot be ignored. We owe it to ourselves, our families, and our patients.

What words or ideas would you offer to help nurses in their career that you wish you'd known?

My nursing career has taken many turns along the way. Initially, I thought I would work in the same hospital for all my career. Now I look back on this journey of multiple departments and several states along the way. It has been a wonderful journey to be part of nursing and to watch it grow.

It took me years to learn to bloom where I was planted. Every change, every department has taught me something about my life and career journey. It has made me who I am. Enjoy the journey. Learn and grow along the way. Never stop learning. Be positive. Have an attitude of gratitude; this has been shown to increase health.

What has been the most rewarding aspect of your nursing career?

The most rewarding aspect I used to think was when I learned to run our rural ED. Then it was managing a medical clinic, passing a rural health survey, learning to deliver a baby, etc. Now it's definitely the fact that I persevered when everyone thought I was crazy in learning these holistic modalities. They laughed when I told them I would start an entire program someday. They scoffed and said, "Never at UMC! It's a county hospital. They won't pay for that." Some of those same people, including physicians, knock on my office door for advice and tools to help them through work, life, and COVID challenges.

We have learned the importance of working together, building each other up, caring for one another. The importance of teamwork. We need each other to get through all of this.

Is there anything else you'd like to share with nurses that could make their lives better?

The importance of self-care is paramount. To be the best you can be, you need to practice techniques that help with stress. Take charge of your health and body. You, your family, and your patients deserve it. It's not selfish to practice self-care. It's imperative. Enjoy the journey. Nursing is a calling, and holistic nursing is a way of being with your patients and your family. It is a way of life.

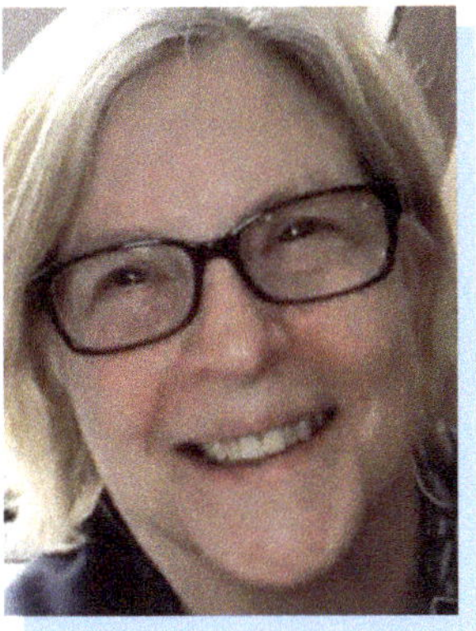

Donna Reagan, MSN, RN

New Jersey

What made you decide to become a nurse? Was there someone or an event that influenced you?

My parents had stopped paying for my education because I didn't maintain the agreed-upon grade point average.

I was waitressing and making good money, so I was deciding what to do next. During this time, I attended the funeral of my grandmother in North Carolina, and my grandfather brought me to visit his father in the hospital before the funeral. During the visit, my grandpa asked me to observe the nurse caring for great-grandad. He said he wanted me to consider this career as an option; he thought I reminded him of this caring nurse. Then at the funeral, my uncle informed me that he thought I was most like my grandmother, out of all of her grandchildren, and because she had been a nurse, I should also be a nurse.

I went home and applied to nursing school. That was thirty-four years ago.

Tell me about your nursing career, such as where you have practiced, what types of facilities you've served in, and how long you have served as a nurse.

I've worked in medical/surgical for two years, then I went to the OR for six years, home care and hospice for about ten years, then back to the OR where I am now. I have completed both my BSN and MSN and am currently in a post-master's certificate program course.

What has been the most challenging aspect of your career in general?

I was most challenged by my orientation and learning how to be a nurse. The other nurses responsible for training me were mean and unsupportive. The burnout was very real to me. Within eight years, I was more than ready to quit; the years of abuse had taken their toll on me.

My career-saving moment came as a flyer in the mail; it announced a holistic nurses' training at Omega Institute. I registered and attended this session, and from the very first moment I entered the room filled with thirty-plus other nurses, I never looked back. This was my tribe, and all that they taught resonated with my soul. Thank God for these nurses!

Do you find the nursing profession stressful? How do you cope with the stress?

Yes, I most definitely find the nursing profession stressful. I now cope with stress through exercise and meditation.

How has the COVID-19 pandemic affected your work?

The pandemic caused me to hustle for hours. I managed to make most of my hours each week. Where I had to work and what I saw was very stressful, but the comradeship of those in the same boat was amazing, and I felt more energized by this than my regular day-to-day practice.

Have there been times you didn't practice self-care when you knew you needed to?

Of course! But things always keep getting worse if self-care is neglected!

What words or ideas would you offer to help nurses in their career that you wish you'd known?

I would say attend to self-care, protect yourself, and avoid overcommitting. Find your tribe and hang with them as often as possible.

What has been the most rewarding aspect of your nursing career?

Finding AHNA and learning about how to care for myself and others.

Is there anything else you'd like to share with nurses that could make their lives better?

Enjoy the moments where you feel connected and journal your experiences. It is very therapeutic to write!

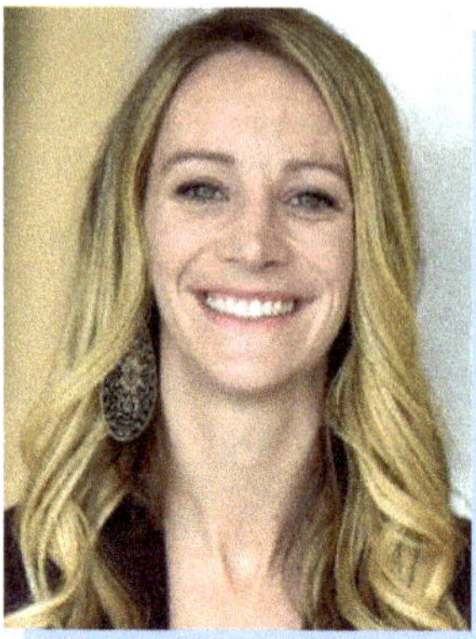

Sara Scheller, RN, Integrative Health Nurse Coach

New Jersey

What made you decide to become a nurse? Was there someone or an event that influenced you?

I was hit by a car when I was four years old, right out in front of my home, while my dad was mowing the grass a few feet away from me. I spent four weeks in the hospital and another ten weeks in a full-body cast from my armpits to my toes. That was an interesting summer, being pulled around in a wagon. Pictures and home videos from the time reflect a happy kid playing ski ball at the boardwalk, riding the pony cars, sitting out by the pool, and blowing bubbles with my sisters. My resilient nature had a lot to do with the caring, loving support from those around me ... especially my mom.

After that experience, I thought I wanted to help people, just like the doctors and nurses helped me. I thought I could be a teacher during the school year, and since teachers get the summer off, I would be a doctor to help the children who got hurt just like me. When I joined medical explorers at a local hospital during high school, a nurse came in as a guest speaker. She said, "Nurses are like teachers and doctors." Well, that was my "aha" moment, and by sophomore year of high school, I knew I had to be a nurse. Quite frankly, it was in my blood as well. My aunt is a nurse and so is my maternal grandmother. My destiny was sealed!

Tell me about your nursing career, such as where you have practiced, what types of facilities you've served in, and how long you have served as a nurse.

I've been a nurse for fourteen years. I was hired right out of nursing school to an ICU internship program. After about three months on a women's health medical/surgical unit, I moved over to the pediatric intensive care unit (PICU). I absolutely loved PICU and worked there for almost five years. I left the PICU when my daughter was about eighteen months old because I was burned out.

To be honest, I was never taught about the importance of practicing self-care, and I became completely overwhelmed with the illness and death I witnessed. On top of that, I experienced role fatigue as a new mom, full-time nurse, and part-time student while I studied for my BSN.

Following my time in PICU, I ventured to the adult cardiovascular intensive care unit (CVICU), where I took care of patients after open-heart surgery. It was completely different from what I was used to. But I learned a lot. In that time, my own heart was broken open as I faced a divorce and learned to stand on my own two feet as I cared for myself and my daughter. I was given/gifted the time I needed to practice self-care when my daughter went with her dad. I found new ways of coping and connecting with my patients.

On top of that, I took a deep dive into understanding more about compassion fatigue, burnout, and self-care strategies. I developed a yearly conference in my health system, called "Nurturing the Nurse," where guest speakers came in to teach a large room full of nurses about nutrition, positive psychology, financial wellness, meditation, mindfulness, resilience, and sleep strategies for shift workers. In between speakers, we practiced yoga, deep breathing, and enjoyed healthy, nutritious food.

I believe in timing, and when someone from our newly grant-funded integrative health and medicine program approached me about a new role they had created, I knew it was time to step out of the ICU and into my full-time role as a health coach.

After about two and a half years in the grant-funded program, I had the unique opportunity to have a more significant impact through corporate nursing education. I now serve as the integrative health coach for our system. This is a dynamic role in which I train and support nurses and others in our health system in providing holistic, complementary, and integrative care to our patients, communities, and each other. I have an ability to affect the nursing practice in our organization through our shared governance model and contributions in writing policies and procedures.

One thing I love about nursing is the flexibility in the profession and all the opportunities available. In nursing, quite literally, anything is possible. With vision, grit, determination, and action, a nurse can create a life they love. Nursing is truly my passion and calling. While I do not have a "traditional" nursing role, I have the ability to touch many lives through my work.

What has been the most challenging aspect of your career in general?

The most challenging time in my career was in my first five or so years as a nurse. I was just shy of twenty-one years old when I graduated, so I was trying to discover who I truly was. I was energetic and passionate about the work, but I didn't have balance in my life. It was depressing to feel burned out at age twenty-five! I didn't like the feeling of counting down the years until retirement; I still had at least forty years ahead of me!

I learned that I could essentially create my own path in life, and then be resilient to how long that might take or precisely what that would look like. I discovered that I didn't have to know everything; I just needed to listen to my heart and lean into my friends, family, and colleagues for support.

Nursing isn't something you do alone. It's a team sport.

Do you find the nursing profession stressful? How do you cope with the stress?

There was a time when I found my work to be extremely stressful. I had trouble sleeping, and I would "check-in" at work to see how my patients were doing. I had a hard time "letting go" of what happened on my shift, and I became anxious about what I would face on my next shift. This is where a mindfulness practice and spending time in nature completely changed my life.

Whenever I noticed my mind wandering, I would bring myself back to the present moment. I began looking forward to sunrises and sunsets, whether on my way to or from work, or watching out the window from a patient's room. I began running, practicing yoga, and spending time connecting with myself and all the beauty around me. The more energy I placed there, the more I recognized my values and my purpose statement.

Some days, I looked in the mirror and committed to making a difference in ONE life that day. Focusing on the moments with my patients and their family members kept me grounded and connected.

How has the COVID-19 pandemic affected your work?

At the start of the pandemic, I was redeployed to support our occupational health COVID command center. It was hard watching the calls come in from nurses and other healthcare workers across our system who were sick. I saw friends and colleagues throughout my health system become sick and even hospitalized with symptoms from COVID-19. That all made it hit home.

Now in the wake of the pandemic, I'm watching many friends from the hospital, where I spent more than ten years, fight for a fair union contract. The public has shown their support for our healthcare heroes, and I hope they're treated fairly as they deserve.

As nurses, we didn't think we were signing up to put our own lives and the lives of our families on the line. Nurses have bravely stepped up to show the tremendous value they offer to our patients and communities.

Have there been times you didn't practice self-care when you knew you needed to?

Of course. If there is one thing we all probably need more of, it's self-care. I don't think self-care necessarily needs to be a big event or even a trip to the nail salon. When I'm feeling overwhelmed, I practice taking three nice big, deep belly breaths. Bonus points if I can stop and close my eyes at the same time. I find that resets and shifts my mind and body, and it doesn't take a lot of time.

What words or ideas would you offer to help nurses in their career that you wish you'd known?

My advice would be for nurses to understand the value of work-life balance. This could look different for everyone and is a highly individualized and personal process. I recommend that nurses spend more time in self-reflection and experiment with different self-care practices to place in their resiliency toolbox. Then, with practice and tapping into your inner knowing, you can reach for the tool you have available or need at that moment.

I also wish I learned more about creating healthy boundaries in my personal and professional life. I found I could relax and enjoy my break when I did a quick set of rounds to my patients and said, "I'm going on my lunch break now, I'll be back at ______________. If you need anything, nurse ____________________ will be taking care of you while I'm gone." My patients appreciated that I was caring for myself and they felt cared for that someone would be looking out for them in my absence. Breaks are not for the weak. They are how the strong remain that way!

What has been the most rewarding aspect of your nursing career?

The most rewarding aspect of my career is looking back and seeing how far I've come. I have not taken a linear path, and I recognize that all the twists and turns along the way have shaped me into the nurse and person I am today. I can look back and say I've grown in giant leaps and bounds.

When I worked with older adults, I loved listening to their stories about life and love. I gained so much wisdom in actively listening and holding the space for them to transform when they told their stories. Nursing has taught me so much about life, and for that, I am extremely grateful. Not even a single day should be taken for granted.

"Sandy," RN, MPH

New York

What made you decide to become a nurse? Was there someone or an event that influenced you?

Years ago, I read a book by George Eliot called *Middlemarch*, and it changed my life. It was so inspirational. To me, what I took from it was finding something meaningful to do, and nursing just hit me. So that's what I did. I've never regretted it. I love it.

Tell me about your nursing career, such as where you have practiced, what types of facilities you've served in, and how long you have served as a nurse.

Oh my gosh. I've been in the nursing field for many, many years. I started as a nurse's aide, and then I went to nursing school. I've worked mostly in nursing homes. I love geriatric care. I feel like I could relate to my residents. I genuinely care about achieving the best outcomes for them. I've done everything up until being a director of nursing. I'm retired now, but I did everything along the way.

My actual favorite job was when I did the education; I was the in-service coordinator and infection-control coordinator. I did a lot of different things over the years. I was a complete workaholic, which nurses tend to be.

Kind of a funny story . . . right before I retired, I had cellulitis and sepsis. I was extremely ill. I'm fine now, thank God. But what was funny is I woke up one morning and had a red circle on my leg, and it was kind of painful, but I went to work anyway. As the day went on, it got worse. Anyway, when I arrived at the ER, finally, I was telling the story to the nurses, and I said, "Well I have this painful red circle on my leg, so I went to work," and they said, "Oh, you must be a nurse." I replied, "Yes, I am. How did you know?" And we all laughed at this well-known nurse behavior.

I had experience working in hospitals, as well as in nursing homes. For about two years, I worked for Indian Health in California, which I really enjoyed. It was interesting and challenging.

I only did ER in nursing school. I went to nursing school in Israel, and it was a different program. We worked the whole way through nursing school. They put us in the hospital so we could work in a variety of settings. We got a good feel for the job and learned so much. During that time, I worked in an emergency room, cardiology, and labor and delivery. I did many different things, and that increased my love for the profession.

The only thing I felt I couldn't do is pediatrics because my heart went out to those children. It was tough for me. Little children don't understand what's going on. You could try to comfort them and soothe them, but with babies, you can't always, so that just broke my heart. That's the one thing I could never do as a nurse.

Many people are called to pediatrics, but it's not for me.

What has been the most challenging aspect of your career in general?

One of the biggest challenges I experienced was as a staff educator, where I worked very closely with the CNAs, and I heard many of their concerns. I realized there's been a shift in healthcare in many places, and unfortunately, it has become more of a money-focused business now. It's much more now than back in the day when it was a little bit more altruistic.

They're cutting staff now, but nurses are still expected to get the job done even without a strong core staff. That's a big challenge, and that's a challenge all the way up. It's a challenge for the CNAs to get their work done. It's also a challenge for management; how do you adequately staff and make sure everybody gets what they need? It's terrible.

Another aspect I want to mention is how we're hiring a lot more per diems, which means it's not a full-time job and lacks benefits. People come to get jobs, and all we have available is per diem. People could be per diem for years. That means they have to work in this place or that place, or wherever they can get work. They're exhausted. They're not getting benefits. They're not fully appreciated. They're feeling blamed for everything, and it's heartbreaking. I'm glad I had a chance to mention that in this book, and hopefully, it'll make a statement.

Do you find the nursing profession stressful? How do you cope with the stress?

At the very end, before I retired, there was a lot of stress because there were many changes in regulations happening. A lot fell on my shoulders since I was doing the education. I wore many hats at the end. And I wasn't feeling well and had a lot of health issues. My children said, "Mom, enough."

To cope with the stress, I was using EFT, which is a form of self-administered acupressure combined with talk therapy for myself. And I taught a few people how to do it at work, which was helpful for them. And I meditate; that's very calming. I also became a vegan a while ago. I'd been a vegetarian for many years, but when I became a vegan, it was wonderful for me. I felt very peaceful. I don't know if you'd call that self-care, but in a way, it is. And it was important to me.

I also try to take a walk every day, and get out in the world, get out in nature. It's relaxing and rejuvenating to take a walk. I'm not a very athletic person, but I do love walking.

Have there been times you didn't practice self-care when you knew you needed to?

I found the night shift challenging, and I was always exhausted. I worked night shift when my children were in high school and thought I'd be more available to them. In other words, when I would be working, they were sleeping; I would sleep while they were at school, and I'd be available in the evening. That was my plan.

However, I was so exhausted that even though my body was there, I'd crash on the couch, trying to keep my eyes open. I mean, it was tough. I know some people love nights and have worked nights for years.

I found it hard to practice self-nurturing because I was just trying to stay awake. I started gaining a lot of weight during those years and was overeating. I don't know if I was actually hungrier or if I thought eating would keep me awake. But I put on a ton of weight. And I began to develop arthritis and all kinds of health issues that might have been connected to working nights or to the stress.

That was a period of time when it was difficult for me to even think about self-care. I was just basically trying to stay awake, be a decent mom, and do my job.

What words or ideas would you offer to help nurses in their career that you wish you'd known?

They should try to remember why they're in nursing and remember that it's a very important job. And when I say nursing, I include nurses' aides and all the aspects of nursing care. It's important not to let your exhaustion turn you against nursing. And to understand that, along with your decision to be a provider of care for your patients, you also have to put yourself on the list of receiving care. Because I know very often, especially women, we take care of everybody else and not ourselves.

As much as you're dedicated to caring for everybody else, you also must remember, if you don't care for yourself, you won't be able to continue doing this work. Remember that if this work is meaningful for you, it's essential to take care of yourself, even if you think you don't have time.

It's not selfish to practice self-care. Many of us think, oh, I don't have time, self-care is not that important, or I feel guilty. But we need to be on that list of people we're taking care of. We are just as important as our patients and our children and our family and our partners and whomever else we're caring for.

What has been the most rewarding aspect of your nursing career?

Oh, wow. There are so many! The feeling that I tried to do some good in the world is important to me.

I remember working with a resident when I was a nurse manager. This resident was a little bit cranky, and she was wearing a beautiful sweater one day. I walked by and said, "Oh, Sylvia, I love your sweater. You look so pretty." All of a sudden, her face brightened up. She said, "Really, you love my sweater. Really? Do you like the color? And does my hair look okay?" It was unbelievable. She was like a new woman. She lightened up, and it was funny and wonderful. It made me realize that every little thing we do affects somebody and can brighten their day.

Even though we might think it's such a little thing to say, "Oh, that's such a pretty sweater," to someone, it struck me how that small act can be important to them. If we just have a smile on our face and speak to somebody and offer encouraging words like "Oh, it's so nice to see you. You look so lovely today," you can really change somebody's life and brighten their day. Since I became aware of her reaction, I now try my best to do that for more people.

Is there anything else you'd like to share with nurses that could make their lives better?

When I taught, I used to remind students and staff members that we all have problems and issues, but when you come to work, try to leave them in your car. You're there to be a loving presence for your residents or patients. Treat the patients the way you would want someone to treat your mom.

Nursing has been such a wonderful and rewarding career for me, and I have such a warm feeling when talking about it. I'm grateful I was able to be a part of it.

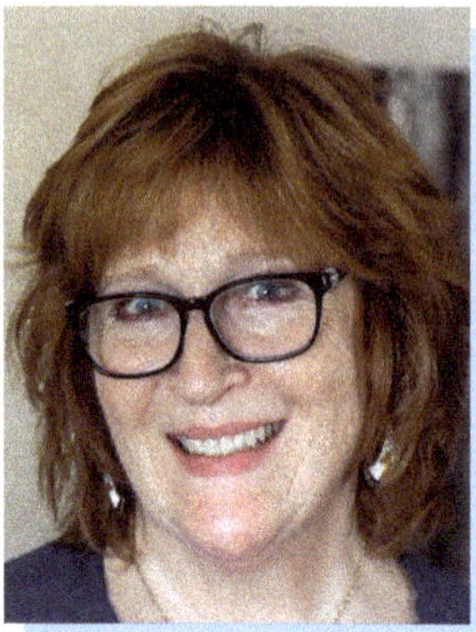

Vicki Crist, RN, LMT

Ohio

What made you decide to become a nurse? Was there someone or an event that influenced you?

It was an accident, but not really; I think the directions our lives take us are often unexpected, while at the same time, we're right where we need and are meant to be. I'm a Jungian advocate, and it's always our unconscious that determines our soul's journey.

I was a very good student, and when I started my education at Ohio State, I had intended to become a veterinarian. But my parents were divorced a year before I graduated, and I experienced a deep depression during my senior year of high school, which resulted in a week of hospitalization in a psychiatric ward. After leaving the hospital, I couldn't get grounded nor focused.

I tried to go to college at Ohio State and dropped out twice. At that point, I came home, went to work, and attended our local community college. I was blessed. The Divine always puts what we need in our path, even if we must trip over it to get our attention.

In my case, it was a beautiful black stallion, who was five years old and as lost as I was. It was a healing journey for both of us. I was twenty-two at the time, had changed my major several times, and realized I needed a major that would provide me with a job paying me enough to buy hay for my beloved horse. My sister-in-law was a nurse and we talked about it, and I knew I could complete the nursing curriculum and get licensed in three years. And so I did.

Having said all that, it didn't take me long to get to know my colleagues, and many of us had grown up being caretakers at a young age. I later explored all those issues in therapy.

Tell me about your nursing career, such as where you have practiced, what types of facilities you've served in, and how long you have served as a nurse.

I practiced nursing at Cleveland Clinic in Cleveland, Ohio. I started in orthopedics for eighteen months, left for a few months, and returned to work in psychiatry; I was recovering from a broken engagement and still a bit depressed, so I thought it only appropriate. Haha. But it was the beginning of the most rewarding time in my career.

I stayed in psychiatry for three years, and it was an interesting milieu—because tucked away on the psychiatric ward were three rooms that housed chronic pain patients. I became familiar with the nurses that worked with the "pain patients," as they were called, and knew it was what I wanted to do.

The Chronic Pain Program, the first in the area, was separate from psychiatry, but it was located there and headed up by Dr. Ed Covington. Dr. Covington was a gifted psychiatrist, a great teacher, and a difficult and challenging man to work with. It was my father all over again; another challenge put in my pathway that forced me to deal with issues of childhood. I stayed there for about fourteen years. I loved the work.

We had our clients for thirty days; we met with them for one hour, three times a week. I led stress management group sessions. I taught meditation and was a coleader for both family group and the dynamic group with Dr. Covington. I also taught assertiveness. It was a multidisciplinary approach to management of chronic pain.

We detoxed our clients off all narcotics and dealt with all psychological issues related to the pain. A holistic approach to managing pain was greatly needed, since most practitioners didn't know what to do with the folks, and it often resulted in a frustrating experience for patient and doctor. Our patients came to us as a last resort after trying many other solutions to their pain. They also did biofeedback and physical therapy.

We treated their depression with medication, which also assisted in alleviating their pain. It was a perfect blend of mind-body medicine. And during that time, I took many counseling courses and started doing my own therapy with a wonderful therapist. This was a rich and rewarding time in my life. As my self-awareness blossomed, I was able to better assist in the healing process and not rescue people—but be a container as they explored their own issues.

What has been the most challenging aspect of your career in general?

This is an easy question. It was so difficult to give patients what they really needed in a hospital setting. I never got involved in management, although I was in a teaching role many times. If I had, perhaps I could have made a difference. But from my experience, the managers who made patients, and their closest caregivers, a priority either left or were dismissed.

Do you find the nursing profession stressful? How do you cope with the stress?

For me, the nursing profession was very stressful, and the best way I found to balance that was taking a different path into more holistic areas. I started in massage school fifteen years into my nursing career. I had the good fortune to study with doctors in oriental medicine and doctors in Traditional Chinese Medicine, as well as many others. I studied Therapeutic Touch with Deloris Kreiger and her students, which led me down the path of Energy Medicine. And I recently received my certification in Emotional Freedom Techniques.

There was one other thing that, for me, was extremely stressful in the healthcare setting. There were situations when patients were harmed by medicines or procedures prescribed for them. There was one time when shock therapy was scheduled for a patient. The night before, the patient asked me about it because he had concerns. He was a young businessman, and this could compromise his memory. He decided not to go ahead with the treatment. As it happened, he had depression and alcoholism and needed help with those issues, not shock therapy. That is where a nurse's role is so important: to always be an advocate for the client and empower them to make their own choices.

Have there been times you didn't practice self-care when you knew you needed to?

Yes, there are still times I don't practice self-care. It's a process. I just get back on track.

What words or ideas would you offer to help nurses in their career that you wish you'd known?

Make self-care a habit. And when you get off track, forgive yourself and get right back on!

What has been the most rewarding aspect of your nursing career?

The most rewarding aspect of nursing was and continues to be being a part of the healing process. I can't think of anything more rewarding and a more spiritual path in life. I always say that if I'm not learning as much from my clients as they are from me, I'm not doing my job. The most important things to me in working with clients are to respect them and meet them where they are, to be open to their experience and respect their choices, to empower them and support them especially in a hospital environment affirm to them that everything is their choice.

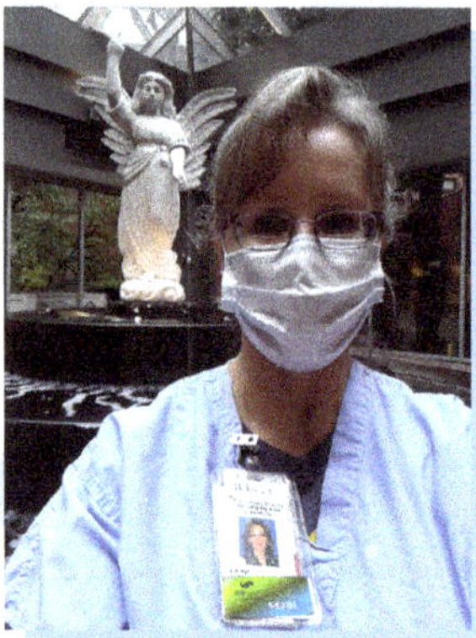
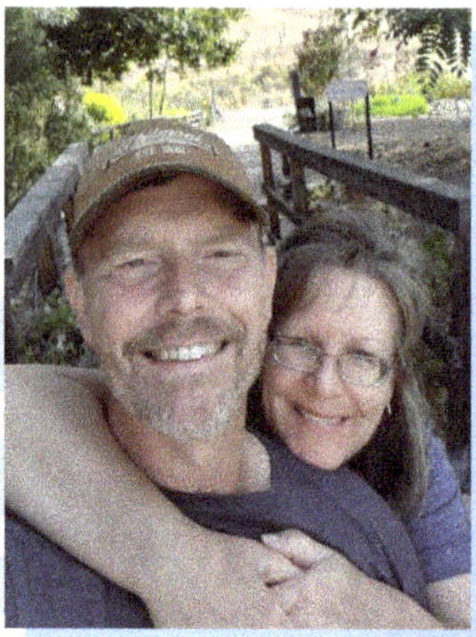
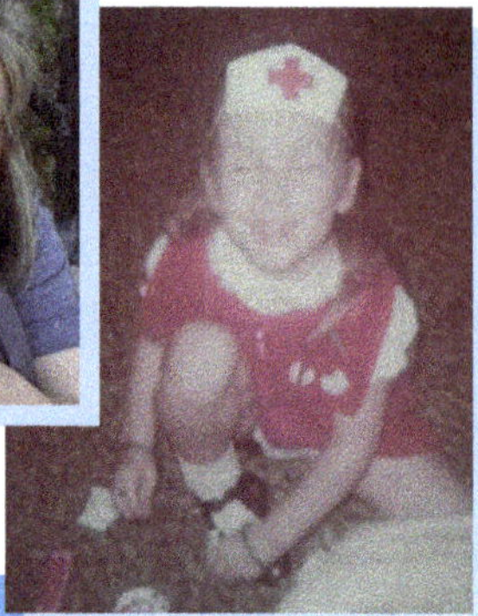

Laurel Gibbs, MSN, MSA, RN, LMT

Oklahoma

What made you decide to become a nurse? Was there someone or an event that influenced you?

My mother was a nurse and I followed in her footsteps. I was intrigued by the way she cared for people and I listened to her stories. When I was a little girl, she would take me into her office, where I would spend the day with her. She'd make a nursing cap for my doll, and my doll and I would spend the day helping my mom.

Tell me about your nursing career, such as where you have practiced, what types of facilities you've served in, and how long you have served as a nurse.

I graduated in December 1992. I started my career in oncology, married, and moved to England, where I volunteered with the American Red Cross on Royal Air Force Lakenheath. I worked for Family Advocacy with the US Air Force, public health in North Dakota, Child Adolescent Partial Hospitalization Program, teaching with various CNA, LPN, and RN programs, office nursing, fetal ultrasound/

counseling, endoscopy, and step-down ICU. I also volunteer at a free medical clinic for an underserved population.

What has been the most challenging aspect of your career in general?

The most challenging aspect has been getting patients to take charge of their own health care, encouraging patients to understand the importance of self-care and the value of their health.

Do you find the nursing profession stressful? How do you cope with the stress?

Yes, most definitely. I want to do so much more but feel limited by time and workload. Two things help me to let go of stress: boundaries and quiet time.

First, by setting boundaries, I'm able to provide patients with information and then let go. They didn't get to this ailment overnight, and I can't fix them in twenty minutes. Second, quiet time takes different forms for me. It might be solitude, gardening, nap time, reading, dancing in the living room, shower/bath, swimming, bird watching, vacuuming, or crafts. It's my time to enjoy, and it's spent reflecting on positive aspects of life.

How has the COVID-19 pandemic affected your work?

I've been furloughed for several weeks and have only recently returned. I am PRN (as needed), so I'm not in the thick of it day-to-day. However, I see my coworkers, and they are stressed. It's such an uncertain time with gray guidelines that seem to change by the hour.

Have there been times you didn't practice self-care when you knew you needed to?

Yes, especially when I was a young nurse out to save the world. My family suffered from my exhaustion, and I suffered from the guilt of feeling torn between work and family time.

What words or ideas would you offer to help nurses in their career that you wish you'd known?

Take time for yourself. You will be better, stronger, happier, and more devoted to life when you feel rested. It can be as simple as treating yourself to an ice cream cone (that you don't have to share with anyone), getting a massage, sitting on a park bench for thirty minutes before you go home, or smelling the flowers in the gift shop or around the hospital before going into work or as you leave. It's so important to be present in your life at this particular moment, and only rest can do that for you.

What has been the most rewarding aspect of your nursing career?

Knowing I made a positive impact in a person's life. Allowing patients to share their medical journey with me and embracing their experience to be a positive one despite the desired outcome. Showing patients that the journey through the process can provide wellness, joy, comfort, and healing from fear. Most importantly, letting them know they've been heard and are valued.

Is there anything else you'd like to share with nurses that could make their lives better?

I think it's important to be kind to each other. Put aside personal judgments, gossip, competitiveness, and let's embrace our individual talents. We each bring a unique gift to our profession, and when we're allowed to share it, the environment becomes richer. If you find yourself in a negative thought about something or someone, be wise as to how you express this thought. Will this thought or feeling bring about harmony, possibly solving the issue, or will it create animosity among others? Be wise with your words, kind in your heart, and recognize when you're not happy/content and make a change. Start with self-care!

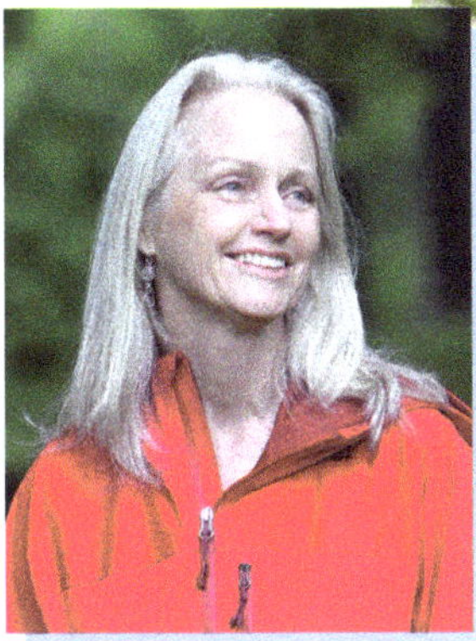
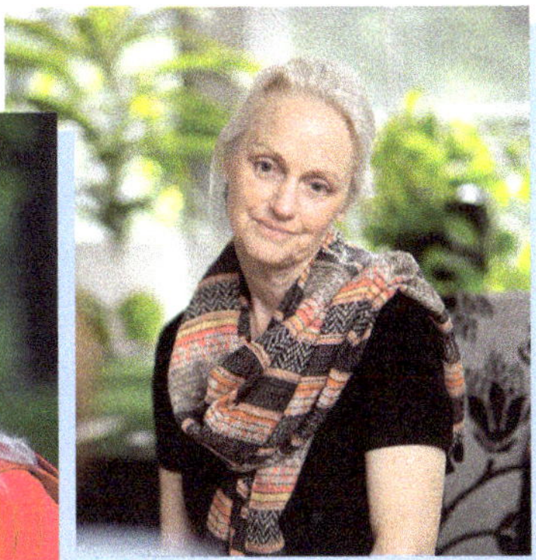
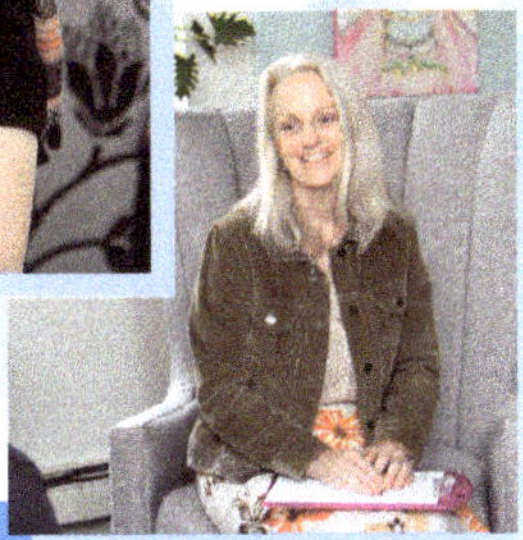

Maggie Brown, MSN, RN, AHN-BC, HWNC-BC, Certified Forest Therapy Guide, Reiki Master Teacher

Pennsylvania

What made you decide to become a nurse? Was there someone or an event that influenced you?

I always enjoyed caring for the elderly, which included my grandparents and great aunts. I also enjoyed being of service, so I decided to become a candy striper at the local hospital. Chatting with the patients and doing simple things, like filling their water or straightening up their rooms, seemed to mean so much to them.

When it came time to go to college, I wanted to follow my true passion: marine biology. However, my father said he would only help me pay for college if I was a nurse, teacher, or engineer. So, I attended a university that had a great marine biology program, and it also happened to be the number two nursing school in the nation at that time.

Freshman year classes were very similar, biology, chemistry, and physics, so I planned to switch to marine biology when my parents weren't paying attention. But then I met my fellow nursing students and the faculty and realized that this might truly be my calling.

Tell me about your nursing career, such as where you have practiced, what types of facilities you've served in, and how long you have served as a nurse.

I've been a nurse for over thirty-three years.

I began in the acute-care setting in an inner-city teaching hospital. I was on a forty-bed medical unit with telemetry, respiratory isolation, and regular medical beds. We were the first unit to get the patients. We also took care of AIDS patients.

We had extremely sick patients and were very busy, and staffing was dangerously low at times. Realizing that many of the patients could have prevented their level of illness with lifestyle changes, I decided to go into primary care so I could support individuals' preventative care. I hoped to find a way to empower people to take control of their well-being, so I obtained my MSN as an adult nurse practitioner.

Again, my desire to be of service directed my next step, and I worked in healthcare for the homeless. The clinic was next to a men's shelter and was an NP-run clinic, which provided a great deal of autonomy for me as a CRNP. The physicians came every other week to review cases and see patients. The richness of this experience came with learning to practice holistically in the most difficult of settings and meeting each patient with unconditional acceptance and compassion.

Next, I worked for the doctors who backed the homeless clinic in their private practice. Even though my patients now had insurance, the major life challenges of wanting to be well, safe, and seen were the same.

The rest of my time as a CRNP came working at an NP-run clinic in a subsidized housing complex in the city. I learned to address/acknowledge complex medical, social, psychological, and societal issues. I decided after having given birth to three children in less than four years, I would take time off to be fully present for them. During this time, I began to explore integrative therapies for myself and my immediate family.

I also began to share what I learned with friends and extended family. I saw that people wanted to be given stress management and integrative wellness tools. And I discovered the AHNA and was pleased to find other nurses of the same mindset. So, I decided to certify as an advanced holistic nurse, a stress management coach, and a health and wellness nurse coach.

Since 2008, I've had a small private practice in coaching,[8] walking beside clients as they discover their path to wellness.

What has been the most challenging aspect of your career in general?

The acute-care setting was most challenging due to inadequate staffing and long shifts. It has been hard to see the role of the nurse practitioner become so focused on the medical model. It has been hard to watch nursing schools let go of the more traditional, integrative approach.

Do you find the nursing profession stressful? How do you cope with the stress?

I found nursing incredibly stressful in the acute-care setting. I also found that the role of the nurse practitioner became more stressful once we obtained prescriptive authority and positioned ourselves as physician extenders. I'm a nurse, not a physician extension. I felt like we sold out the very essence of nursing to make more money and market ourselves.

I also began to have my patient time slots triple booked. All this was very stressful, and I was exhausted. Plus, I had a new marriage and a young family during these years, so there was no wiggle room for self-care.

When I began to see my children picked up last at daycare all the time, I acknowledged to myself that this was one of the biggest stressors. So, I left my job and took a "time out." I began learning integrative therapies while I spent more time with my children.

Now I'm a health and wellness nurse coach. I never book my clients back to back, because I want time to extend the appointment if needed, to chart, and energetically clear the room for the next client.

I work part-time to allow for self-care. I put aside the notion handed to me as a young person that my worth as a human was dependent on the work that I did. No longer was working "so hard" a badge of honor.

I appreciate this quote from His Holiness the Dalai Lama, "Man surprised me most about humanity. Because he sacrifices his health in order to make money. Then he sacrifices money to recuperate his health. And then he is so anxious about the future that he does not enjoy the present; the result being that he does not live in the present or the future; he lives as if he is never going to die, and then dies having never really lived."

How has the COVID-19 pandemic affected your work?

I've been the lead organizer on a not-for-profit project called The Compassion Caravan.[9] It was an amazing project that was to launch May 10, 2020, in New York and ending in New Mexico in June 2020. I remember that at the AHNA 2019 conference, I started talking to Terry Maluk about this. I was so inspired to meet her and to sit next to someone who was living and traveling in an RV. The traveling seemed doable. The vision became clearer: a project of traveling while offering compassionate listening circles, self-care education, forest therapy, and creating a thread of connection along the way.

Below is an excerpt from an interview I did with Heidi Rodgers, editor of the research newsletter for the AHNA:[10]

> *When I shared my vision, people would say "this is a great idea", and "this is so needed." So, I reached out! I reached out to nursing theorists for their blessing. At first, I thought it would just be a few nurses involved, but a lot of holistic nurses came forward with their resources and wanted to volunteer their thoughts, enthusiasm, and expertise to create a beautiful program. I reached out to The Omega Institute for sponsorship for retreat space, and they said, "Yes! We want to sponsor you!" With great enthusiasm, many other people came together to*

support us. The artist, Gaia Orian, designed the image for The Compassion Caravan, and i123 donated web support. Individuals concerned about the well-being of nursing stepped forward in donating time. Dr. Helen Erickson and Margaret Erickson, CEO of the AHNCC, were incredibly supportive and created a beautiful program of mobilizing self-care resources through offering an expressive art self-reflection as a part of the workshop. With the help of a core group of holistic nurses from AHNA Chapters, the Compassion Caravan project blossomed into a national project that offered the power of compassionate healing presence, interconnectedness, and integration.

So, we were ready to rock and roll and all the things were in place, and then COVID-19 hit and we were detoured. We detoured into the virtual world and now we are holding virtual Compassionate Listening Circles. These are becoming their own thing and are very meaningful for the people who are participating.

Mindful self-compassion training really informs the Compassionate Listening Circles and I would love to see this become a component of nursing education. Hopefully the misnomer of "compassion fatigue" will disappear. It's empathy fatigue, not compassion fatigue, that nurses are experiencing.

Our Compassionate Listening Circles are now being held 3 times per week. There is a Nurses in Nature Retreat planned for October, but the COVID-19 numbers are going up, so we will see. Since it is a "wait and see" at this point, I am going to take a "time out" from a lot of doing. We are kind of in a waiting pattern, so I am going to devote 40 days of meditation to support the unfolding during this unknown. I picked the day of the new moon to begin my "time out" (July 20th) and I counted 40 days out, and it ends on my son's birthday, my son who passed . . . that is so interesting to me.

COVID-19 has been a challenge to my private practice; it is hard to market classes and gatherings when we sit in such unknown.

Have there been times you didn't practice self-care when you knew you needed to?

Definitely. Working the night shift in the acute-care setting. I did seven months straight of nights, and it hit me hard physically, emotionally, and spiritually. I was just plain exhausted. It wasn't good for my body, and I was too tired to practice self-care.

What words or ideas would you offer to help nurses in their career that you wish you'd known?

"No" is a sentence. You don't have to explain yourself for not taking on extra shifts. You are no good to your patients if you're exhausted. I took on a lot of night shifts so I could pay off my college loans quicker, which wasn't really in my best interest.

It took me a while to figure out that I could choose my own path in nursing. There was a lot of the "oh, she is not a 'real nurse'" kind of thing if you weren't overworked, which is so silly.

What has been the most rewarding aspect of your nursing career?

Getting to walk beside people on their journey here on Earth. The appreciation of bidirectionality and interconnectedness.

Is there anything else you'd like to share with nurses that could make their lives better?

Practice self-compassion and loving-kindness toward yourself. If you're not sure how to develop these skills, reach out to someone who's trained to support you in this endeavor. It will provide a pathway to living with ease.

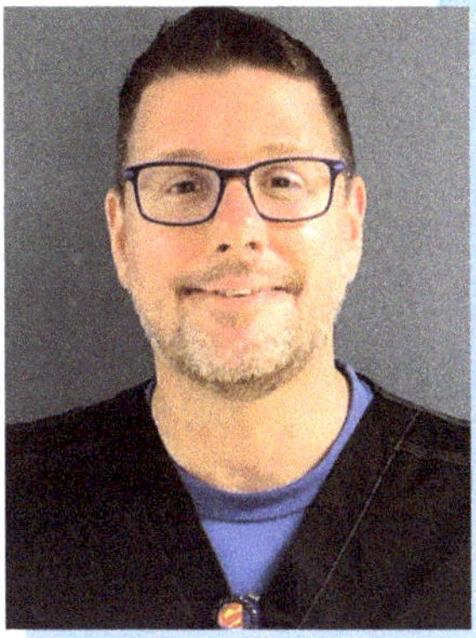

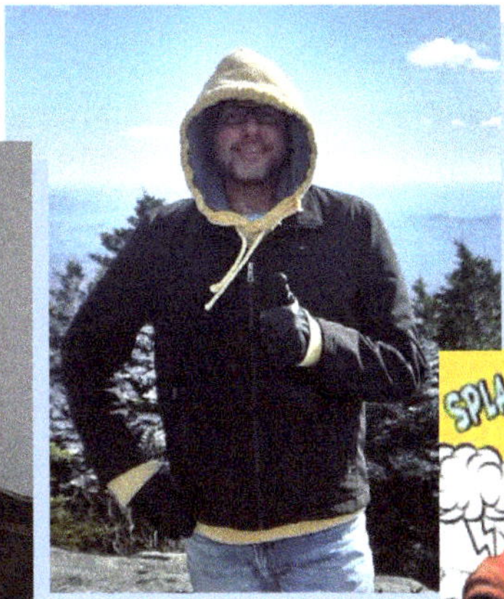

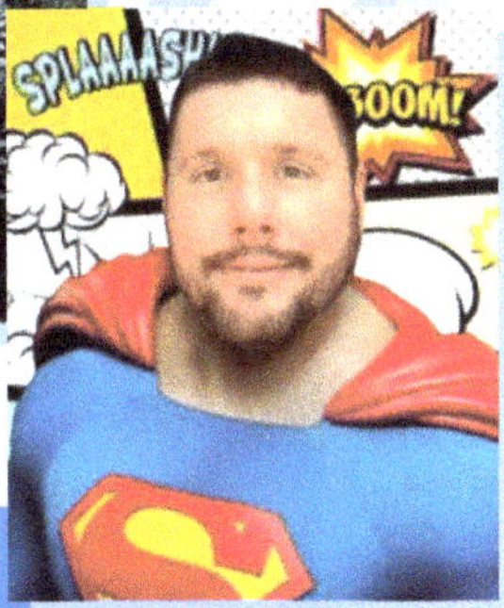

Craig Metcalf, MSN, RN

South Carolina

What made you decide to become a nurse? Was there someone or an event that influenced you?

I gave thought to entering nursing school and becoming a registered nurse (RN) during my twenties. Still, even back then, I had enough insight into my own being to know that I didn't have the "stick-to-it-iveness" to maintain the discipline and determination to see it through. Nursing school, in and of itself, requires an incredible amount of time, energy, and organizational skills, and those just weren't my strong points during my earlier years. When I was in my late forties (yes, I'm a "late bloomer" to the nursing field), I truly felt ready and able to commit to the rigor, the stresses, *and* the rewards of a nursing career. More specifically, it was my training in mind-body practices, such as yoga and meditation, which helped me to reach that point; those disciplines have integrated beautifully into my nursing practice. They have helped me to become a more holistically-minded RN, which is something I strongly feel benefits my patients as well as their family members.

Tell me about your nursing career, such as where you have practiced, what types of facilities you've served in, and how long you have served as a nurse.

I hold a master of science in nursing (MSN), and I'm an experienced registered yoga teacher (E-RYT). In addition, I am certified through the American Heart Association as a basic life support (BLS) instructor.

My healthcare career began while still in nursing school, when I obtained my certified nursing assistant (CNA) and was hired as a personal care attendant (PCA) within an acute care center through one of the community's local healthcare organizations.

After graduating with my associate degree in nursing (ADN) and obtaining my nursing licensure, I transitioned into my RN role on the same unit, which was a step-down telemetry unit, serving adult populations. My entire experience there lasted approximately two years, and I reached a point where I wanted to branch out and see what other nursing opportunities and experiences were available.

Since leaving the hospital, I've had the opportunity to transition into pediatric nursing roles, which have been amazing experiences. From serving as a transportation nurse, working one-on-one within a local school district and serving children with special needs, to serving as a pediatric private duty nurse through home healthcare, the journey has been incredible. I am in my fourth year of my nursing career and look forward to many more.

What has been the most challenging aspect of your career in general?

I suppose the most significant challenge, during the first two years or so anyway, was learning to integrate nursing knowledge with critical thinking skills. A nurse must not only know, for instance, what a given lab value generally means. He or she must also be able to apply that knowledge in holistic ways to the patient's specific situation, condition, and needs; this helps to ensure the best possible patient care and patient outcomes. And that skill takes time and practice to develop and improve.

Do you find the nursing profession stressful? How do you cope with the stress?

Yes, I used to, much more so when I worked in a hospital. Again, my training in yoga and meditation helped me manage stress more effectively, and I'm incredibly grateful to have acquired those skills. Nowadays, in my current nursing capacity, stress levels are much lower, and I'm extremely grateful for that, too!

Have there been times you didn't practice self-care when you knew you needed to?

This probably occurred more often during my first year of nursing while working in a hospital setting. Over time, I've made self-care a priority, and now it's a daily habit.

What words or ideas would you offer to help nurses in their career that you wish you'd known?

You owe it to yourself, as well as to your patients, to take care of yourself. Self-care will not only save your physical and mental well-being, but it can also help reduce such things as medication errors, workplace aggression, and the ability to think critically during medical emergencies. This is because you've already taken good care of yourself, which places you in a much better position to practice patient care to a higher level of integrity.

What has been the most rewarding aspect of the nursing career?

It's when I have the opportunity to apply a little "psych nursing" to patient care. Beyond skill sets, such as successfully starting an IV, inserting a urinary catheter, or assisting with a paracentesis procedure, one of the greatest rewards of nursing comes from connecting with patients on an emotional level. When a patient is having a difficult time adjusting to a given diagnosis, or when they're lonely and upset because their family has left them behind . . . those situations are, in my opinion, *specifically* suited for nurses to engage.

For me, there's no greater reward in my career than helping someone through that rough time and letting them know that I'm there and will try my best to help in whatever ways I'm able. This isn't to say that nurses are saints. I, myself, recognize that I can be self-absorbed and perhaps even a little self-centered at times. We are human! But, overall, I do feel that nurses are naturally drawn to this profession because of its ability to expose us to unique situations, which offer us a chance to practice a different kind of healing, beyond the physical aspects of patient care.

Is there anything else you'd like to share with nurses that could make their lives better?

Why do, as the old saying goes, nurses "eat their young"? Even within today's more culturally responsible health care arena, some experienced nurses still treat new nurses with a fair amount of disdain, disrespect, and just flat out bullying. Why do such nurses engage in that type of behavior and choose to create an environment of fear and intimidation? From where does that mentality spring forth?

I experienced it during my first year of nursing, and I know others who've had to endure similar experiences. Some might consider it to be a "rite of passage" of sorts, but I personally think it embodies the antithesis of what it means to be a nursing professional. I'll admit, I don't have any concrete solutions to this issue, but the nursing profession, as a whole, ought to be delving more into this culture of fear and aggression and asking itself, "How can patients and other health care disciplines trust us and take us seriously if we can't even trust or take seriously those within our own ranks?"

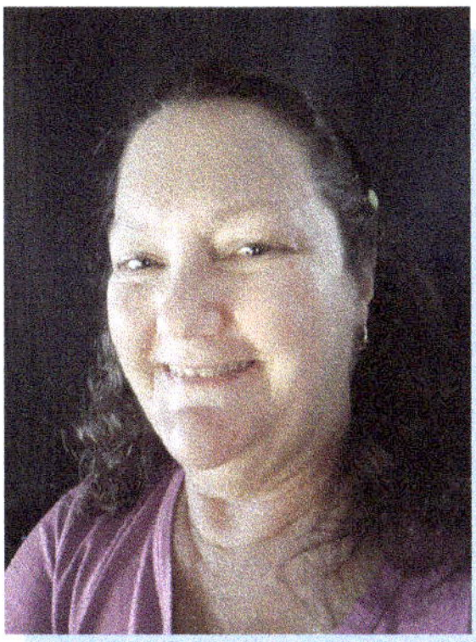

Kathi Bury, RN, BSN, CPN, MSCAM, Certified Aromatherapist, Reiki Practitioner

Texas

What made you decide to become a nurse? Was there someone or an event that influenced you?

I've wanted to be a nurse since I was a little girl.

Tell me about your nursing career, such as where you have practiced, what types of facilities you've served in, and how long you have served as a nurse.

I've been a nurse for twenty-six years. I started as a floor nurse in a federal prison hospital and then moved to a county public-health clinic. After this, I discovered that I liked emergency medicine, and in particular, pediatrics. I stayed in pediatrics until I couldn't do bedside nursing anymore.

What has been the most challenging aspect of your career in general?

Being assaulted by patients and families. The implication that I had to work while sick or risk being penalized. Never being able to take a break for meals.

Do you find the nursing profession stressful? How do you cope with the stress?

Very stressful. I think I internalized it all and ignored my body's stress signals and ended up with bulging discs in my back and chronic pain. Now I meditate, take deep breaths, and use aromatherapy to help with stress. I also stopped working at the bedside.

How has the COVID-19 pandemic affected your work?

I now do pediatric telephone triage from home. I've been doing this for about eight months. The pandemic hasn't really affected my work. But it has affected my life in other areas, such as not going out for groceries and other things, and I've had to reduce contact with my son and his family because he's a firefighter and is constantly exposed to the virus. I miss them and the hugs tremendously.

Have there been times you didn't practice self-care when you knew you needed to?

Always when working, because it was never allowed. There were penalties for taking sick days. We had to take up the slack when there was insufficient staff, assistance, or equipment. I was also counseled once because I was kicked in the face by a patient and injured; the message was that if I complained about an injury, I'd be treated like a whiner and mentally compromised.

What words or ideas would you offer to help nurses in their career that you wish you'd known?

ALWAYS put yourself before the job! No employee isirreplaceable. They'll take everything you have, wring you out and keep on going, leaving you in the dust. You're more important than the job. Pushing yourself beyond your comfort zone and being a martyr only benefits the employer. Meanwhile, you're the one hurt by allowing yourself to be taken advantage of.

What has been the most rewarding aspect of your nursing career?

I love working with children. They have no agenda. They just want to feel better. They are sweet and loving and tremendously giving. They always made my heart happy to spend time with them. That was why I pushed myself so hard.

Is there anything else you'd like to share with nurses that could make their lives better?

Treat yourself as you would treat your patient. Never expect yourself to work under conditions that you wouldn't want your best friend to work under.

Sandy, RN, BSN

Unnamed State

What made you decide to become a nurse? Was there someone or an event that influenced you?

In high school, I didn't know what I wanted to do. My mother raised four children by herself, so we didn't have very much money. My aunt in Atlanta offered to pay for me to go to nursing school. I hadn't thought about that. I went up one week to Atlanta and I interviewed at Piedmont Hospital, which was a three-year diploma school. Then my aunt took me to Emory University, but back in the day, it was five years to become a nurse at Emory.

I kept thinking . . . five years or three years? So, I ended up going to Piedmont. I graduated from nursing school in 1963. We worked as well as went to school back then. We worked more than we were in school, but it was a wonderful experience. I wouldn't trade anything for it.

My aunt paid $350 for my schooling at Piedmont. She would have picked Emory University, but I just couldn't get my head around five years in school.

I received an excellent education at Piedmont College. I ended up getting a BSN later. I gained a lot of practical experience, which went a long way toward getting your first job. Because when you graduate, you're pretty much ready to work.

Tell me about your nursing career, such as where you have practiced, what types of facilities you've served in, and how long you have served as a nurse.

Well, my first job was at Piedmont Hospital, and it was medical/surgical. I was young and single, so I didn't stay there long. I was there when Kennedy was shot. Then, I briefly did a little psych nursing. It was interesting enough, but I didn't really take to that.

Then I moved to a 900-bed big city hospital in Flint, Michigan. I worked in intensive care, which was interesting, and I learned a great deal. It was a wholly different experience from the private hospital where I went to school. The people that we saw in the intensive care area in the city included a lot of trauma and gunshot wounds and the whole nine yards. I learned a ton and enjoyed it, except I'm a people person and many of the people weren't able to speak. I decided at that point, even though I liked it a lot, it wasn't what I wanted to do.

Back in those days, every year and a half or so, I moved to a new place. From there, I went to Johns Hopkins and worked in the recovery room. They called it the PACU. They would also take intensive care patients, and that was a phenomenal learning experience for me. The nurses that worked there were also very inspiring. At Johns Hopkins, there was heart surgery, and I'd never been around heart patients, and they did a lot of neurosurgery. It was just incredible.

They also did tonsillectomies, and back then, they used ether. Patients couldn't be discharged until they drank something. When patients came back to recovery, they'd feel awful, and they were nauseated. We'd have to try to get these little three- and four-year-old children to drink.

After Johns Hopkins, I went to Savannah and went to work at a hospital, and I got married to my high school sweetheart. The small hospital in Savannah was so impressed with the experiences that I had.

My husband was going to finish his studies at the University of Georgia in Athens, so we moved to Athens. They asked me if I'd like to be a day supervisor. I was only twenty-three or twenty-four, but I agreed to do it. It was another good experience because I had a work background that they'd never had. I remember walking into this patient's room, who had had a tracheotomy, and they had suction, and the suction tube was just lying there. They weren't thinking about contamination. There were several things that they were not doing but should be doing. It was good to bring what I had learned to this new job, things that really helped the hospital and the patients too.

They had two OBs at Athens General Hospital, one for paying patients and another OB for non-paying patients. In each one would be a nurse supervisor and an LPN. At the time, they had three doctors who worked in the emergency room, and one of those doctors would come to deliver the baby, but half the time, the doctor wouldn't come, because of emergency room duties. So, the LPN and I delivered forty babies in the two years I worked there. For the most part, they were people who had more than one baby, so it was a whole lot easier to deliver again.

I taught them how to improve colostomy care. I realized at that time that I probably could teach if I wanted to, because I enjoyed it. At my last job, I was the only person who would take students willingly. I always felt like if I could impart what I know, I've done my job and helped them.

New students have a lot of knowledge, but they lack the practical experience. I've had so many people come back to me over the years and say, "You don't know how much you meant to me and what you gave me."

After we left Athens, Georgia, we went to New Orleans, and I worked at a hospital there in the SDU (step-down unit), and I liked that because you could talk to people.

Right now, I'm working at an eye surgery center. My job is to call the patients ahead of time and get their health histories and list of medications and tell them which medicines they should take and what people with diabetes should do with their insulin. It's great fun for me because most of the people love getting the phone call since they don't have many other people to talk to.

What has been the most challenging aspect of your career in general?

To me, it was the doctors. A lot of them made life hard for nurses, and some doctors didn't respect the nurses.

Another frustrating thing was trying to affect change. Trying to be honest about how things could be made better, but then nothing would ever change.

In one job, when I was prepping patients for surgery, my boss said, "You know what needs to be done. You design the process that you know will work." That was a thrilling and wonderful experience being able to set it up efficiently, and then when I retired, to pass it over for the next person to use and make their own improvements.

Do you find the nursing profession stressful? How do you cope with the stress?

The most stressful thing was the sheer volume of things I had to do to get a patient ready for surgery, and I had three patients to get ready at the same time.

To cope with the stress, I'd go home and walk six miles, and I'd feel like a different person. Or I'd ride my bike. I rode my bike across the country from San Diego to St. Augustine. They put a map of my route on the wall in my unit to track my progress.

Even with all the stressful times, though, I wouldn't have changed being a nurse.

Have there been times you didn't practice self-care when you knew you needed to?

I've got to be honest; I remember being stressed out, but taking a little bit of time off was all I ever needed.

As a young nurse, we had a lot to do, but the types of cases weren't as severe as they have now. I don't know how nurses today do it with five or six really sick patients at a time. It's just different now. It doesn't seem like hospitals care about their nurses.

What words or ideas would you offer to help nurses in their career that you wish you'd known?

Join your nursing organization and create a power base so that you can change things. That's the only way things will change, and it takes a lot of effort. Stand up for smaller nurse/patient ratios.

Don't be afraid to seek help when you need it, whether from a therapist or taking up a hobby totally separated from the hospital so you meet new people.

Get enough physical exercise, like walking or biking outside.

Speak up because the key to lowering stress is to have fewer patients to take care of. Nurses today are overwhelmed. People always say it's a money thing, but you have to keep nurses happy, or they're going to leave the profession.

What has been the most the most rewarding aspect of your nursing career?

The most rewarding part about my career has been helping change people's lives for the better in small incremental ways that are little effort for me but mean a lot to them.

Nurses can do small things, like touching the patients gently, sitting by them, and letting them tell you about their life. Being able to talk with patients and give them my time was very rewarding, plus showing respect to people no matter their background. To me, that's what it's all about—taking care of them, helping them get well, and helping them know how to take care of themselves when they're discharged. All that falls to a nurse. To be honest, I can't think of another job that's so meaningful.

Is there anything else you'd like to share with nurses that could make their lives better?

One of the things that I'm also passionate about is a basic four-year degree for nurses. Doctors have consistent levels of education. Nurses' education needs to be standardized as well. Currently, we have LPNs, RNs, and BSNs working, and it all should be standardized.

And it's crucial to participate in and give back to your community.

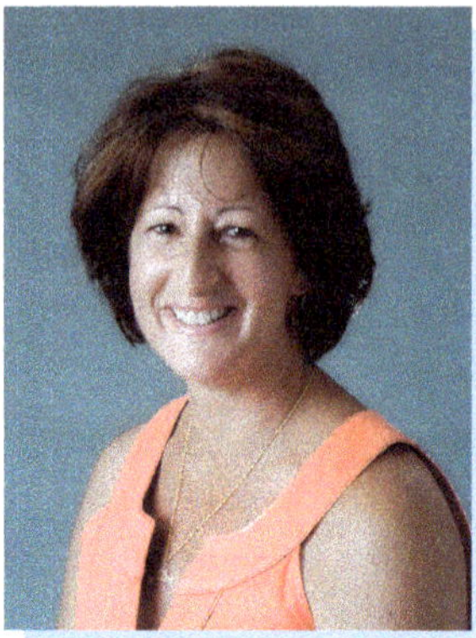

Ann Cowper, RN, BSN, HNB-BC

Virginia

What made you decide to become a nurse? Was there someone or an event that influenced you?

My mother was a nurse, and as one of two females in my house, we were only encouraged to have traditional female roles; I am a nurse, and my sister is a teacher. I remember being fascinated by the machines and activities when I would pick Mom up from work and visit the ICU. As it turns out, I am a healer, so I guess it was the path for me.

Tell me about your nursing career, such as where you have practiced, what types of facilities you've served in, and how long you have served as a nurse.

Although I have been in healthcare since I was fifteen years old, I have worked as a nurse since 1985. My first experience was in neuroscience and neuro ICU at Massachusetts General, where I learned how to be a nurse and about advanced medicine. I worked at the Medical College of Virginia in Richmond at a neuroscience ICU, but it was a very bad experience, and so I left.

I also worked in a medical ICU, then in case management, and care coordination when it was first being developed and showed cost savings. I also have experience in home health and community health nursing in a low-income community clinic. I started a nutrition business somewhere in the middle and continued that for a few years until I had a stroke.

Now, after ten years of recovery, I am re-emerging as a holistic health coach and working on certification for nurse coaching. I am proud to be a certified holistic nurse, where I learned to embrace nursing. Nurse coaching is helping me heal from my nursing experiences and as a wounded healer archetype.

What has been the most challenging aspect of your career in general?

To be honest, the most challenging part of my career and my life has been working with other health professionals and nursing professors. I started out very naïve, and I've never been very conventional, so I didn't feel that I fit in.

I will never forget the first nurse that taught me how to be a nurse; it was in my first job. She was angry but honest. She said I was doing it all wrong, and she was right! It wasn't the way they taught me in nursing school. Through interactions with many angry nurses and doctors, I've learned to be strong and know myself.

When I had a stroke, I had to learn to stick up for myself in the health profession and get what I needed that would support me. I would say that I have come full circle.

Do you find the nursing profession stressful? How do you cope with the stress?

The nursing profession is very stressful. That seems obvious to me. But we have to learn to work within our abilities and not expect more than we can produce in a day. I remember in my later years, telling myself, "If I don't have time to finish this paperwork, who has time to read it?

I think I will trim it back because the most important part of my work is the connection with my patients."

Also, we have to understand that we don't "owe" our patients better health. We can only be present to offer it and accept their response. We should honor ourselves. Now I have the healthcare providers that support my personal health care, and I'm working confidently with nurses in the holistic field.

How has the COVID-19 pandemic affected your work?

Fortunately, I am not in the inpatient setting any longer. Restarting my professional coaching practice began in January 2020, and I was hoping to remarket locally, but when the pandemic hit, I turned online and learned a lot. Teaching the public about the disease, inflammation, and correcting misconceptions became exhausting after a couple of months, and I went offline for a while. Like many people, I'm making real changes in my life and finding out what is mine to teach. I'm confident, like many, that I will emerge a happier person.

Have there been times you didn't practice self-care when you knew you needed to?

Part of my changes involved leaving a relationship that has compromised my self-care and the work I love. It's been a couple of years in coming. The challenge has been in over-caring for the other person and rescuing them to the point of exhaustion. I'm looking toward recovering and bringing this to my work. It's hard to watch someone you love deteriorate. I'd learned a long time ago to accept people where they are, help those who want it, and send compassion to the rest, but this one caught me off guard.

What words or ideas would you offer to help nurses in their career that you wish you'd known?

Remember that as a nurse, sometimes you're a healer, sometimes you're a teacher, and sometimes you're a technician, and that is okay. Take the time to find your authentic self and your place in the healthcare system. There's room for everyone. And support each other. Whenever you feel angry toward another nurse, recognize they're only bringing up something in you that needs to be healed. Have compassion, patience, and confidence in yourself that you'll eventually figure it out.

What has been the most rewarding aspect of your nursing career?

Hands down, the most rewarding part of nursing is when I'm working with a client who begins to find their own way. They make changes and get healthier and happier, and I'm just there to cheer them on!

Is there anything else you'd like to share with nurses that could make their lives better?

My wish for nurses is that we begin to collaborate more and recognize our power in numbers to make changes in the healthcare system, nationally and internationally.

Gretchen Schodde, MN, ARNP, FNP-BC, NC-BC, Founder & Executive Director Emerita of Harmony Hill

Washington

What made you decide to become a nurse? Was there someone or an event that influenced you?

I was always interested in being a healthcare professional. When I learned that the future of nursing would include nurse practitioners, I signed up.

Tell me about your nursing career, such as where you have practiced, what types of facilities you've served in, and how long you have served as a nurse.

Initially, I was a public health nurse, including home visiting. Then I became one of the first family nurse practitioners in a rural area in Washington State as the movement was starting in the early 1970s. I practiced in a remote clinic with one other nurse mentored by two MDs thirty miles away. We had significant support via the University of Washington (UW) School of Nursing.

I returned to UW to participate in the development of the Nurse Practitioner Master's program. I joined the faculty for seven years with a focus on outreach to rural and underserved areas. Later, I taught assessment skills at two community colleges.

In 1985, I moved to Union, Washington, and founded Harmony Hill,[11] a retreat center focused on healthy living for all, and to provide transformational retreats for cancer patients and their caregivers.

I also became an integrative nurse coach and joined the faculty to provide programs at Harmony Hill. I'm also on the leadership team for the Commonweal[12] Nurse Leadership for Healing Circles, providing a learning community for people with cancer and those who care for them.

What has been the most challenging aspect of your career in general?

Fundraising is always a challenge for the programs I run at Harmony Hill. The funds are needed to provide our three-day cancer retreats at no cost to participants.

Do you find the nursing profession stressful? How do you cope with the stress?

Mostly I have loved being a nurse—and yes, it's stressful at times. I cope with stress by being with colleagues as we gather in healing circles, by gardening, and being in nature.

Have there been times you didn't practice self-care when you knew you needed to?

Yes, I often work long days, and I'm still learning to stop and refresh more often.

What words or ideas would you offer to help nurses in their career that you wish you'd known?

Regular check-ins with colleagues who are role models for self-care. Also, finding and practicing stress reduction and healthy living tools, such as meditation, gentle exercise, healthy nutrition, and a daily gratitude journal.

What is the most rewarding aspect of the nursing profession?

The heart-and-soul work with patients we serve, and inspiring colleagues with whom I provide healing services.

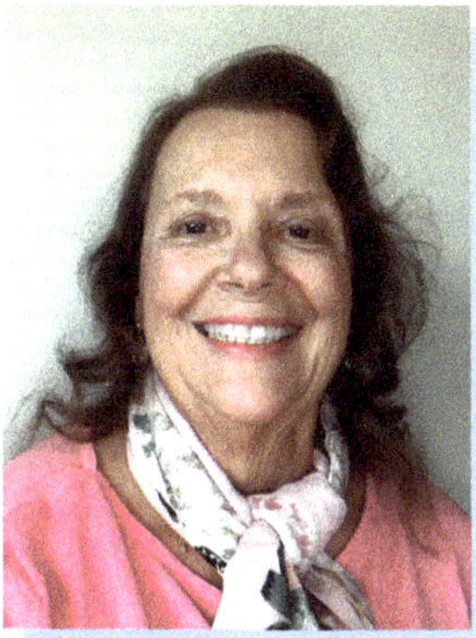

Linda Kathleen Morton, RN, MBA

Washington

What made you decide to become a nurse? Was there someone or an event that influenced you?

My grandmother raised me, and from as little as I can remember, I was always told I'd be a nurse. At that time, when I was growing up in Montgomery, Alabama, women didn't have a lot of options. You could study to become a schoolteacher or a nurse, or if you couldn't go to school, you could become a secretary, or you could be a homemaker. Those were the only opportunities that we had, at least in my circle of reference. My aunt was a teller in a bank, but she only did that as more of a fun job so she could have spending money, not as a career. There were not many single, family women raising children.

As long as I can remember, back in the 1950s, my grandmother and I used to go to the library, and I'd always pick out all the nursing books to read about it. I'd bring them home, read all of them, and then we'd go back to the library. So, I was spoon-fed everything about nursing from the time I was very, very small. When I fell in a bike accident and was hospitalized with a severe infection, I saw a nurse's work. Frenchy was a nurse at Jackson Hospital and had a tremendous influence on me. My cousin Patty Bloodworth was a brilliant RN who should have been a physician.

At that time in Montgomery, there was a prominent Catholic hospital there, St. Margaret's, which had the only nursing program. You didn't have bachelor's degree programs for nursing then. Nurses, typically in the South, went to a hospital and were trained by the nuns, very stringently. They graduated and became nurses, usually at the same hospital or another hospital around town.

When I was fourteen, I went to my church, Capital Heights Baptist Church, and asked if they'd pay for my nurse's aide class and my first set of uniforms. So, I went to work in a hospital at the age of fourteen, and I've been in healthcare ever since then.

And here I am at seventy years old and retired. So I've seen ups and downs and everything that could possibly happen in healthcare in my fifty-six years of service.

Tell me about your nursing career, such as where you have practiced, what types of facilities you've served in, and how long you have served as a nurse.

While I was in Birmingham, I went to school at Jefferson State Nursing School and earned my associate degree in nursing. When I graduated from nursing school, it was a big deal to me to excel. I was president of the Alabama Nurses Association while I was in school. I traveled to all of their meetings. I graduated and got special training in NICU because ICU at that time was the top echelon for nurses. I went to work in ICU. I worked in cardiac ICU, medical ICU, neuro ICU, and later on in surgical ICU.

When I got burned out from that, I went to work in the recovery room. And then, I left the recovery room and went to Shepherd Spinal Hospital in Atlanta (now the Shepherd Center) and worked mainly with newly diagnosed teenagers in their ICU that had spinal cord injuries.

I've worked in so many departments. I worked in medical review for Blue Cross Blue Shield and worked with providers all over Georgia supporting physicians in their practices. I have worked in healthcare consulting for clinical support as a liaison between nursing and information technology on computer implementation and support for Kaiser.

I moved back to Columbus, Georgia, where my mother lives, and I couldn't find a nursing job, except for night shift. So, I went to work at Blue Cross Blue Shield of Georgia, first in medical review, and then I became a manager of all their coding unit. I had over 100 employees. I worked with a vice president there who gave me a chance. He had come from IT, and he and I worked together and developed a program to do online coding for Blue Cross Blue Shield.

While I was working in Columbus for Blue Cross Blue Shield, I earned my BSN degree. And I got my master's degree while working full time at Catholic Health Initiatives. I was the manager of all of their clinical and business applications for hospitals.

I got interested in informatics, and I did that for about four years. Then I went to work in Provider Relations at Blue Cross Blue Shield in the processing of claims and learning how doctors' offices operated with claims coding and all that. I traveled all over the state of Georgia and went to doctors' offices from Columbus. My territory kept growing until I had about half the state. At that time, I was offered a job from Blue Cross Blue Shield of Oregon, to go out there and supervise their Provider Relation Liaison Team for the whole state of Oregon. That brought me to the Pacific Northwest.

I always worked while being a mother and wanting to excel. I always worked a part-time job on the weekends. When I was in Columbus, I did psych nursing in a psychiatric facility. Then when I came out to Oregon, I worked weekends in the surgical ICU. I met my husband and moved to Eugene, Oregon. Blue Cross Blue Shield didn't have a facility there. So I went to work at the local hospital, first in nursing triage over the phone. With the computers, you work with computer programs, and then I became their liaison between nursing and IT. That brought me to Seattle because I got an opportunity to work for a software company. And from there, I went into consulting.

I've also worked in public health nursing. Later on in life, I moved to Moses Lake, where I was the Manager of Public Health for Grant County. And then, toward my retirement, I became a school nurse and worked for the Washington Extension Office, teaching nutrition in underprivileged schools that had a lot of immigrant children.

What has been the most challenging aspect of your career in general?

I think for nurses in general, shift work is very, very difficult. The nursing aspect and the care of the patient are what brings the most joy. But in some hospitals, they have rotating shifts. Shift work isolates nurses to a great extent. They're isolated from their family and their friends. And the night shift is very, very stressful because the most horrible things happen at night in the hospital when there are very few support systems in play. I'd say that's the most stressful.

I worked night shift in the ICU at one point. I was the only person in the entire hospital, including the supervisors, that could interpret the readouts from the monitors connected to the patients. That meant I couldn't even go to the bathroom without fear that somebody would have tachycardia or something, and I wouldn't be there to see it. So, I had no meal breaks, no breaks at all. I was literally working the entire time I was there. And night shift is stressful on the body, physically, because you're trying to sleep when everybody's awake, and the phones keep ringing. It's difficult.

Do you find the nursing profession stressful? How do you cope with the stress?

In the early years, I didn't cope very well. I'd do things like come off night shift and drink a few glasses of wine before I went to sleep. A lot of nurses take Benadryl or some other sleep aid. You don't really get a good night's sleep when you're doing that sort of thing.

In my later years, when I had to go in, I'd usually just stay up until I could go to bed in the evenings and then sleep on my regular pattern. I'd just be very, very tired.

I found the most comfortable shift to work was 3:00 p.m. to 11:00 p.m. because you still had your morning. You were working late, but you could still come home and go to bed and sleep and wake up and have a portion of your day.

Have there been times you didn't practice self-care when you knew you needed to?

Yes, definitely. In the early days, I think nurses as a whole didn't practice self-care. They cared for other people. So, they would do a lot of self-destructive things. They would smoke cigarettes. They'd get in destructive relationships. They would drink heavily. I think nurses are very codependent, and in being codependent, the most important thing is to learn to take care of yourself first and then take care of other people.

What words or ideas would you offer to help nurses in their career that you wish you'd known?

A lot of managers guilt people into taking on more work, even when they know the person doesn't need it or is exhausted. They guilt them into it. "You're the only one I can rely on. I can always count on you." Those words to a codependent are music to their ears. If they think their patients won't receive proper care if they don't stay, then they're going to stay.

In many ways, learning to take care of yourself is not taught in nursing school. You're taught to take care of others, but you're not learning how to take care of yourself.

Also, it's okay to say, "I don't know that," or "I'm exhausted," or "I don't feel comfortable doing that." All those are great skills for nurses to learn. Or "I need some more skill-building on that. You're asking me to put in a PICC line, and I've only done one before, and it was three years ago." It's okay to speak up and say those things.

The other thing I think is challenging is that most management people in nursing have risen through the ranks. They've not been taught; they haven't gone to college and learned management skills and how to manage people and how to grow people. So the bad traits are passed on, such as guilting people into coming in for that extra shift. If you're a good manager, you plan for staffing shortages, like during holidays. Those are things that need to be taught, too.

If you look at a lot of nurses, they're overweight, they're stressed out, and they're in bad emotional relationships. If nurses could exercise and eat better, practice more self-care, both they and their patients would be so much better off.

What has been the most rewarding aspect of your nursing career?

While working in the inpatient setting, there was one man who was so depressed, he was just starving to death. One other nurse and I decided to keep him alive. We played radio music, and every night we'd come in and say, "It's time to party," and we got him eating again. It was a special time. She was a fantastic nurse.

When I worked in ICU, I loved to take patients that no one else wanted. I remember I took a stroke patient one time that was unconscious. I talked to his wife and said, "We need to exercise his limbs." I'd sit by his bed and talk to him during my shift and tell him what I was doing and why I was doing it. And I told his wife that she needed to try to get him into the best rehab facility that she could. He was eventually moved out, and about six months later, that man came to the door of ICU where I worked, and he walked in and said, "You saved my life. I know you don't know it, but I heard every word you said to me."

I love nursing. I love mentoring people, and I love letting nurses know what an important job they're doing. Nursing is not just a job; it's a passion.

Is there anything else you'd like to share with nurses that could make their lives better?

If people go into nursing for just the money, they're going to find they couldn't be paid enough sometimes to do some of the jobs they're asked to do. I think you've got to have in your heart a love for people. And that's what makes a difference. It's a career where you'll never have a boring day. It's a career to last a lifetime. I treasure those that paved the way for me, and I hope I've made a difference for the patients and families I have served.

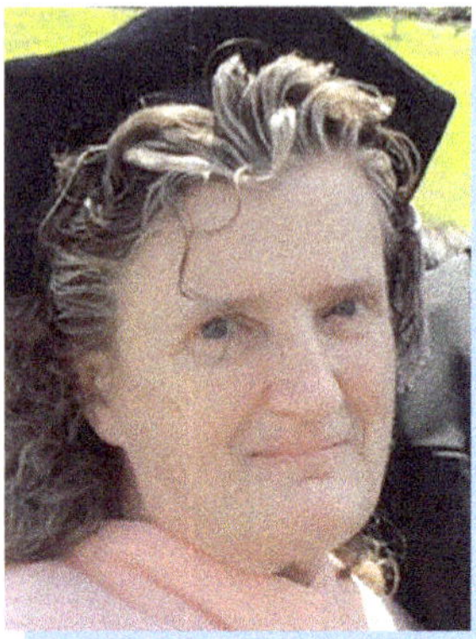

Denice Reese, APRN, DNP

West Virginia

What made you decide to become a nurse? Was there someone or an event that influenced you?

I was an extremely shy person in my late teens and early twenties, and I love science, so I thought being a research biologist would be an ideal career for me. A friend in college, Mike Konstan, who is now a renowned physician and professor in pediatric pulmonology, suggested that I might like to join him volunteering at Rainbow Babies and Children's Hospital. I did, and that changed my life.

We both volunteered with the cystic fibrosis patients, and this experience steered me toward a career in nursing. Those kids lit me up! The following summer, I volunteered at CF camp, and when I returned to campus in the fall, I changed my major. I was close enough that I was able to complete my biology degree, and then I completed my BSN the following year. The shyness evaporated as my confidence grew. I had found my calling, and I have never looked back!

Tell me about your nursing career, such as where you have practiced, what types of facilities you've served in, and how long you have served as a nurse.

My first job as a nurse was in a pediatric intensive care unit at Rainbow Babies and Children's Hospital in Cleveland, where I worked for a little over a year. I transferred to the pediatric emergency room in the same hospital and worked there for another seven years. I loved it so much that I can remember sitting at a stoplight on my day off, wondering what was going on at work and wishing I was there.

Upon moving to West Virginia in 1987, I began a sixteen-year stint as the only school nurse for rural Tucker County, serving four school sites and about 1000 students any given school year. I earned my MSN and became certified as a pediatric nurse practitioner in 1996.

From 2003 to the present, I have taught at Davis & Elkins College, where my specialties are pediatric nursing, pharmacology, and simulation facilitation. I completed my doctorate in 2016, where I did research on online education in Quality Improvement methods. I have done extensive volunteering with migrants in El Paso, Texas, which has been some of the most soul-satisfying work I have ever done.

What has been the most challenging aspect of your career in general?

I have loved being a nurse. The challenges come when there are conflicting priorities and scarce resource allocation.

But the other challenging aspect is my own expectations, which leads to overdoing things and being a workaholic and being very detail-oriented. While these traits have resulted in being a good nurse, they also result in being consumed by work frequently. This has distracted me, at times, from attention to my family and myself.

Do you find the nursing profession stressful? How do you cope with the stress?

Implied in the nursing role is a great deal of responsibility. When involved in direct care, nurses are constantly assessing, analyzing, synthesizing, problem-solving, advocating, and working with others who have different responsibilities and, many times, different priorities. On top of all that executive and collaborative functioning, there are the documentation requirements and the mundane, time-consuming things. Interestingly, in my experience, the least stressful thing is the actual care of the patient. That is where the flow happens and where the focus of caring lifts a lot of stress away.

For the last eighteen years, I've been a professor of nursing at Davis & Elkins College. Now the subjects of my "care" are my students, primarily. Teaching and nursing at an essential level are all about supporting people to achieve their highest potential. The emotional satisfaction of teaching is very similar to the emotional satisfaction of caregiving. Stress arises from all the things that are not directly related to nurturing. Meetings, documentation, and politics are the things that I find the most stressful in this position. And, of course, when students don't pass a class, I'm really sad for them.

So, what do I do to cope? Setting good boundaries is a good start. As a professor, I try to identify a downward trend in a student and give them all the support I can, whether academic or emotional support. Knowing that you have gone the "extra mile" and made yourself available eases feelings of unreasonable hyper-responsibility. I guess, for me, the bottom line is to build all professional actions on a foundation of excellence. And within the foundation, I can feel less stressed.

How has the COVID-19 pandemic affected your work?

The pandemic resulted in all our classes going online. Over a three-day period in March, we pivoted to a very different and significantly less personally satisfying mode for delivering the content of our courses. I teach online in the RN to BSN program and created those classes to be online classes and love teaching them, but turning an in-progress, in-person class with clinical components into an online offering was very labor-intensive and profoundly unsatisfying.

I really missed the emotional satisfaction of connecting with students in the classroom and clinical situations. I missed working in person with my colleagues. All the unknowns made things very hard and very lonely. I finally got in a little better shape mentally by deliberately reaching out to talk with and visit with people on a regular basis. The pandemic has been very disequilibrating.

And in addition to work-related things, there is the personal worry for self and family and others. I am sixty-four years old with some probable risk factors, and thinking about going back to the classroom in the fall is causing a lot of anxiety. I'm thinking about the potential for bad outcomes and wondering if I have my ducks in a row. Sobering stuff indeed.

Have there been times you didn't practice self-care when you knew you needed to?

Absolutely! And much to my own detriment! I tend to get consumed by my work, and the day passes and I haven't taken care of my needs like exercising, stretching, eating healthily, and having fun. Lately, I've been creating a more deliberate way to track the health-promoting and joy-inducing things that I know will result in my well-being, and it has been working!

What words or ideas would you offer to help nurses in their career that you wish you'd known?

I'm not sure this is what I wish I'd known, but rather what has worked for me. I feel like I've had a good attitude for most of my career. I've maximized the roles I've held. I have always found joy in work by really embracing whatever agency I had in the situations where I worked. I built good working relationships where trust and mutual respect were the goals. I've seen a lot of people become disempowered and bitter in their work, and I guess I would say to do whatever you can to avoid that. Don't stay in a job that leaves you empty and frustrated.

I would also say learn what you can in difficult situations and try to influence them for the better, but if you can make no headway, try something else. There are so many things we can do and ways we can serve as nurses. Every moment gives you another chance to have a positive impact on your patients and your coworkers. Bring curiosity, willingness to be a helpful coworker, humor, and love to work with you every day. And don't be pulled down by disempowered people who are entertained by the petty dramas of the work world. I know I sound like a Pollyanna, but someone once said to me, "Yeah, you're a Pollyanna, Denice, but you have your army boots on." I embrace that sentiment.

What has been the most rewarding aspect of your nursing career?

The opportunity to be with people in their most vulnerable moments has been intimate and rewarding. I feel like I was never afraid to be present in those hard moments.

As a teacher, I've found it incredibly rewarding to watch my students blossom in their careers and maximize their impact on the world. As teachers, we are force multipliers! I hear from students all the time saying that they can hear my voice in their heads when they're thinking things through or making decisions. I feel alive in their work. They are my heart and hands going forth into the future. Can't beat that!

Is there anything else you'd like to share with nurses that could make their lives better?

Thanks for the opportunity to share a little about what has been a rich and rewarding career. I can attest that keeping your heart wide open and your spirit generous are gifts that keep on giving, to your patients, their families, and your coworkers, and also to yourself. Gratitude for being in such a role is a good posture to adopt.

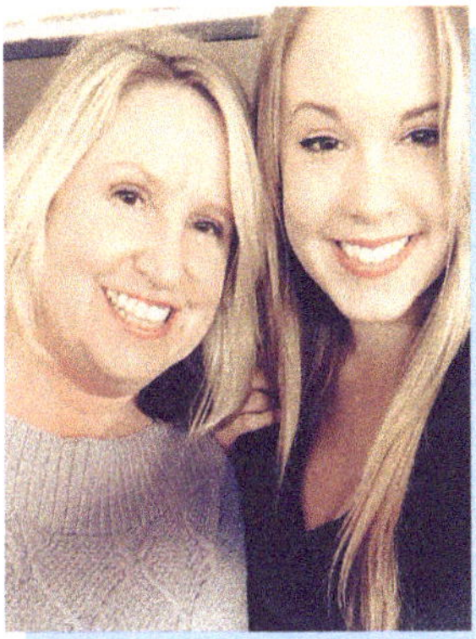

Karen Hartz, BSN, RN, CCRN

Wisconsin

What made you decide to become a nurse? Was there someone or an event that influenced you?

When I was around ten years old, my older cousin was hospitalized for mono. We went to visit her, and I was fascinated with the hospital, nurses, doctors, and just the overall professionalism showed. From that day on, nursing was what I wanted to do.

Tell me about your nursing career, such as where you have practiced, what types of facilities you've served in, and how long you have served as a nurse.

I entered college in 1971, and there were only a handful of universities offering the BSN degree in Michigan. Due to that, I went to Northern Michigan University in Marquette. It was over 550 miles from home, so it was a significant lifestyle change only getting back home maybe two or three times a year.

Upon graduation, I started working at Marquette General on the medical/surgical floor. It was a 400-bed regional hospital, so it was very busy, and I learned a lot. After two years, I switched to ICU, and that has been the love of my life. I moved to the Detroit area in 1978 and worked in ICU at a 500-bed teaching hospital for eighteen years. I moved to Wisconsin and continued to work in numerous ICUs at small regional hospitals.

Currently, I have worked at the same place for twenty-two years.

What has been the most challenging aspect of your career in general?

Balancing professional life with home life. Between raising two children, moving to different states, and going through a divorce, it wasn't easy. I'm blessed, though, because my career has kept me centered and sane through it all. But there are times when I feel torn between my personal life and work life.

Do you find the nursing profession stressful? How do you cope with the stress?

It is stressful. There are always new policies and guidelines to follow. In ICU, there's so much to keep competent on, such as new equipment, medications, and ways to treat all critical illnesses that come our way. Probably the most significant stressor for me is feeling I don't have enough time for my patients and going home wishing I could have done more!

I cope with stress at work by having great camaraderie with my coworkers and with laughter. At home, I take long walks and work in my yard as much as possible and, of course, enjoy an occasional glass of wine.

How has the COVID-19 pandemic affected your work?

Thank goodness we have not seen a large number of positive patients here yet, though daily, the numbers are rising. I experienced two older patients die from COVID-19, and their families could not be at their sides, only talking on a baby monitor through the glass! This did have an impact on me because I've always prided myself in helping families and their loved ones deal with the death and dying process. I find it so sad.

Being in a high-risk category at the age of sixty-seven, I don't give direct patient care to the COVID-19 positives or rule outs. I understand the policy but feel guilty for placing this on my younger colleagues. Overall, there's an atmosphere of fear and frustration with this virus, and it certainly has been the biggest disease entity I have ever experienced in my forty-plus years of nursing!

Have there been times you didn't practice self-care when you knew you needed to?

Definitely. I just kept plugging on when tired and weary and trying to hold things together when my personal life was falling apart. On my days off, I learned to take care of me, but that took years to feel okay with. I now advocate for calling in for a "mental health" day and nap all day if you want. Nursing is wonderful but can destroy you if you're not careful. I have personally watched it happen in my career.

What words or ideas would you offer to help nurses in their career that you wish you'd known?

That you're only one person! Nursing is a 24-7 job. If you don't have the time to complete everything, there's the next shift coming on. Please, please don't feel guilty about handing off things to the next nurse! I'm also a huge advocate for our young nurses starting out. I'm proud to say I've had the honor to precept over fifteen-to-twenty senior nursing students to ICU, with many getting hired after graduation. I detest the concept of "eating our young" and have been very verbal about not tolerating it.

What has been the most rewarding aspect of your nursing career?

It has changed focus over forty-plus years. It used to be whatever it takes to save them, meaning tubes, dialysis, open heart surgeries, pain, and, unfortunately, loss of dignity for life. Now, my most rewarding aspect of nursing is death with dignity and guiding the family and patients through the process. Another rewarding aspect has been teaching and working alongside our young, new awesome nurses!! Very rewarding!

Is there anything else you'd like to share with nurses that could make their lives better?

Be compassionate and treat your patients how you would want your loved ones treated! Take time out for yourself to decompress and experience joy around you.

Acknowledgments

FOR THE MANY wonderful people in my life, words of thanks are hardly enough. I am extremely grateful for you and everything you do.

Lori Snyder, author, writing coach, cheerleader, yoga teacher, and extremely kind person. Thank you for reigniting this project as the COVID-19 pandemic interrupted the nurse interview process and the whole world's sense of normalcy. Thank you for your vision, ideas, and continual encouragement.

Dawn Husted, editor, author, camping enthusiast, and extremely patient person. Thank you for helping me understand a little more of the Chicago Manual of Style with each book, and for answering my last-minute questions right up to the end. Your edits are always relevant and thoughtful.

Laurie Young, designer, user experience guru, and self-proclaimed karaoke queen. Your genuine interest in this project was evident from the first time we spoke. Thank you for intuitively knowing where I wanted to go with the design, and for your skill in artistically highlighting the nurses and their stories.

Emmi Mooney, best friend ever, retired ER nurse, beta reader, reviewer, and artist. I could write a whole book about the times you've lifted me up, inspired me, and supported me as I ventured out of my comfort zone with your encouragement. Thank you for always being there, listening as I vent, and helping me remember how lucky I am.

Connection with family can become so much stronger during challenging times. Thank you to my husband Wes, sisters Cathy, Rosanne, and Deb, daughter Sarah, and granddaughter Emmy for your unceasing love, understanding, support, and encouragement. Through multiple quarantines, sanitizing, distancing, and a serious paucity of hugs, I love you to the moon and back.

Endnotes

Page 12 Introduction

[1] New England Journal of Medicine, https://www.nejm.org/doi/full/10.1056/NEJMp2012114

Page 18 Susan M. Gillispie

[2] Wholistic Health & Wellness, https://www.wholistictelehealth.org/

Page 36 Jessica Brown

[3] Worthy Beyond Purpose, https://www.worthybeyondpurpose.com/

Page 40 Pamela McDonald

[4] APO E Gene Online Program, https://apoegenediet.com/

Page 44 Mary Ann Osborne

[5] Institute for Integral Health, https://instituteforintegralhealth.com/

Page 56 Kim Evans

[6] Institute for Integrative Medicine, https://www.integrativemedicine4u.com/

Page 59 Evans

[7] Evans, Kim. *Transforming Healthcare: Healing You, Me, and Our Broken Disease-Care System*, Butler Books, 2019. https://www.butlerbooks.com/transforming-healthcare.html

Page 127 Maggie Brown

[8] Inner Light Recovery, https://innerlightrecovery.com/

Page 128 Brown

[9] Compassion Caravan, https://www.compassioncaravan.com/

[10] Heidi Honegger Rogers, DNP, FNP-C, APHN-BC. American Holistic Nurses Association, Connections in Holistic Nursing, Volume 12, No. 3, August 7, 2020.

Page 149 Gretchen Schodde

[11] Harmony Hill, https://www.harmonyhill.org/

[12] Commonweal, https://www.commonweal.org/program/hcc/

Appendix:
Stress-Management Resources

"If your compassion does not include yourself, it is incomplete."
—Jack Kornfield

One of the questions asked of the nurses in this book is:

"Do you find the nursing profession stressful?"

As expected, the responses were almost unanimous. The first words of their answers often included, "Yes!" "Of course!" and "Absolutely."

One reason I wanted to collect these stories from nurses who are experiencing and dealing with stressful situations was to let other nurses know they're not alone in their feelings, and that there's hope. I reached out to those who know first-hand what it's like and to share how they cope: advice *from* nurses *for* nurses.

Since the grim reality of the COVID-19 pandemic, nurses have been under fire on the front lines of medical facilities, showing up and doing the best they can in far-from-ideal conditions. Some of the nurses in this book discuss the impact the pandemic has had on them and their work.

What happens when you take a known stressful profession and add an exponential level of stress from a virus whose symptoms and recommended procedures were changing multiple times in a shift? The potential for burnout and secondary trauma suddenly becomes very real.

Chapter 1 of my book *Rx for RNs* talks about stress in the nursing profession:

> *"Nurses tend to be caregivers by nature. Nurturing, altruistic, and compassionate, nurses can be selfless to the point of self-neglect. It's ironic that while nurses have a crucial role in taking care of everyone else, nurses often put their self-care last. Over time, this leads to exhaustion, feelings of overwhelm, and burnout, which helps no one.*
>
> *The nonstop demands in the environments where most nurses work may not always support self-care. Sometimes it's even hard to take time for a bladder break! But it's important to take self-care seriously if you want to continue being of service in such a high-stress profession.*
>
> *Honoring basic needs such as taking the time to use the restroom as needed, so you're not afraid of staying hydrated, having time to enjoy a healthy meal or snack, and taking periodic breaks to pause, take a slow breath, and regroup should be the norm, not the exception . . ."*

There are widely known and accepted sources of information about stress and self-care, and the nurses in this book have suggested several more. This appendix includes a few selected books and websites for further information. This is in no way an exhaustive list but merely a first step as you discover ways to reduce stress and its impacts.

Books

Harris, Dan. *10% Happier: How I Tamed the Voice in My Head, Reduced Stress Without Losing My Edge, and Found Self-Help That Actually Works--A True Story*, Dey Street Books, 2014.

Kabat-Zinn, Jon. *Full Catastrophe Living (Revised Edition): Using the Wisdom of Your Body and Mind to Face Stress, Pain, and Illness*, Bantam, 2013.

Kabat-Zinn, Jon. *Wherever You Go, There You Are: Mindfulness Meditation In Everyday Life*, Hachette Books, 2010.

Maluk, Terry. *Emotional Freedom Techniques: The Art of Managing Stress Through EFT Tapping*, From Stressed To Calm, 2020.

Maluk, Terry. *In This Moment: The Art of Managing Stress Through Meditation*, From Stressed To Calm, 2019.

Maluk, Terry. *Rx for RNs: A Step-by-Step Guide to Manage Stress, Reduce Overwhelm, and Conquer Burnout*, From Stressed To Calm, 2018.

Maluk, Terry. *Take One Breath: The Art of Managing Stress Through Mindful Breathing*, From Stressed To Calm, 2019.

Nagoski, Emily. *Burnout: The Secret to Unlocking the Stress Cycle*, Ballantine Books, 2019.

Sapolsky, Robert M. *Why Zebras Don't Get Ulcers*, Holt Paperbacks, 2004.

Scala, Elizabeth. *Stop Nurse Burnout: What to Do When Working Harder Isn't Working*, Heritage Press Publications, 2016.

Scott, S.J., and Davenport, Barrie. *Declutter Your Mind: How to Stop Worrying, Relieve Anxiety, and Eliminate Negative Thinking*, CreateSpace Independent Publishing Platform, 2016.

Sheridan, Carmel. *The Mindful Nurse: Using the Power of Mindfulness and Compassion to Help You Thrive in Your Work,* Rivertime Press, 2016.

Sweeney, Monica. *Let That Sh*t Go: A Journal for Leaving Your Bullsh*t Behind and Creating a Happy Life*, Castle Point Books, 2018.

Sweeney, Monica. *Zen as F*ck at Work: A Journal for Banishing the Bullsh*t and Finding Calm in the Chaos*, Castle Point Books, 2019.

van der Kolk, Bessel. *The Body Keeps the Score: Mind, Brain and Body in the Transformation of Trauma*, Penguin, 2014.

Websites

American Heart Association – Stress Management: https://www.heart.org/en/healthy-living/healthy-lifestyle/stress-management

American Holistic Nurses Association – Stress Management: https://www.ahna.org/Home/Resources/Stress-Management

American Institute of Stress – http://www.stress.org/

American Psychological Association – Stress relief is within reach: https://www.apa.org/topics/stress

American Psychological Association PsycNet – Mindfulness-Based Stress Reduction for Health Care Professionals: Results from a Randomized Trial: https://psycnet.apa.org/record/2005-05099-004

Emotional Freedom Techniques – The Gold Standard (Official) EFT Tapping Tutorial: https://emofree.com/eft-tutorial/eft-tapping-tutorial.html

From Stressed To Calm – Say Goodbye to Stress: https://fromstressedtocalm.com/

Greater Good Berkeley – Stress: https://greatergood.berkeley.edu/tag/stress

Harvard Health Publishing – Relaxation techniques: Breath control helps quell errant stress response: https://www.health.harvard.edu/mind-and-mood/relaxation-techniques-breath-control-helps-quell-errant-stress-response

Healing Touch – Healing Touch Program: https://discover.healingtouchprogram.com/htp-home

HeartMath – Stress Facts: https://www.heartmath.com/blog/health-and-wellness/stress-facts

Help Guide – Stress Management: https://www.helpguide.org/home-pages/stress-management.htm

National Association for Holistic Aromatherapy – Natural Remedies for Anxiety and Stress: https://naha.org/

Patient Safety & Quality Healthcare – Joint Commission Portal Addresses Nurse Burnout: https://www.psqh.com/analysis/joint-commission-portal-addresses-nurse-burnout/

US National Institutes of Health website articles about stress –

- Stress and hormones: https://www.ncbi.nlm.nih.gov/pmc/articles/PMC3079864
- The Effect of Diaphragmatic Breathing on Attention, Negative Affect and Stress in Healthy Adults: https://www.ncbi.nlm.nih.gov/pmc/articles/PMC5455070
- Effects of the transcendental meditation technique on trait anxiety: a meta-analysis of randomized controlled trials: https://www.ncbi.nlm.nih.gov/pubmed/24107199
- 5 Things You Should Know About Stress: https://www.nimh.nih.gov/health/publications/stress/index.shtml
- The value of mindfulness meditation in the treatment of insomnia: https://www.ncbi.nlm.nih.gov/pubmed/26390335
- Brain Mechanisms Supporting Modulation of Pain by Mindfulness Meditation: https://www.ncbi.nlm.nih.gov/pmc/articles/PMC3090218

University of Michigan Medicine – Stress Management: Breathing Exercises for Relaxation: https://www.uofmhealth.org/health-library/uz2255

Glossary

ADL
Activities of Daily Living

ADN
Associate Degree in Nursing

AHNA
American Holistic Nurses Association

AHN-BC
Advanced Holistic Nurse Board Certified

AHNCC
American Holistic Nurses Credentialing Corporation

APHON
Association of Pediatric Hematology/Oncology Nurses

APO E gene
Apolipoprotein E gene

APRN
Advanced Practice Registered Nurse

ARNP
Advanced Registered Nurse Practitioner

BLS
Basic Life Support

BSN
Bachelor of Science in Nursing

CCRN
Critical Care Registered Nurse

CCU
Coronary Care Unit

CF
Cystic Fibrosis

CMT
Certified Massage Therapist

CNA
Certified Nursing Assistant

CNAT
Certified Nurse Aid Trainee

CNL
Clinical Nurse Leader

CNO
Chief Nursing Officer

CNS-BC
Clinical Nurse Specialist Board Certified

COVID or COVID-19
Corona Virus Disease Originating in 2019

CPHON
Certified Pediatric Hematology Oncology Nurse

CPN
Certified Pediatric Nurse

CRNP
Certified Registered Nurse Practitioner

CVICU
Cardiovascular Intensive Care Unit

DNP
Doctor of Nursing Practice

ED
Emergency Department

EFT
Emotional Freedom Techniques

EKG
Electrocardiogram

EMS
Emergency Medical Services

ER
Emergency Room

E-RYT
Experienced Registered Yoga Teacher

FAAN
Fellows of the American Academy of Nursing

FNP
Family Nurse Practitioner

FNP-BC
Family Nurse Practitioner Board Certified

FNP-C
Certified Family Nurse Practitioner

HIPPA
Health Information Privacy Protection Act

HMIP
HeartMath Interventions Program

HBN-BC or HNB-BC
Holistic Nurse Baccalaureate Board Certified

HPI
History of present illness

HTCP
Healing Touch Certified Practitioner

HWNC-BC
Health and Wellness Nurse Coach Board Certified

ICU
Intensive Care Unit

IV
Intravenous

IT
Information Technology

KHNA
Kentucky Holistic Nurses Association

LL (AAN)
Living Legend of the American Academy of Nursing

LMT
Licensed Massage Therapist

LPN
Licensed Practical Nurse

MBA
Master of Business Administration

MD
Medical Doctor

MICU
Medical Intensive Care Unit

MN
Master of Nursing

MPH
Master of Public Health

MSA
Master of Health Service Administration

MSCAM
Master of Science in Complementary and Alternative Medicine

MSN
Master of Science in Nursing

MSPH
Master of Science in Public Health

NC-BC
Nurse Coach Board Certified

NCCA
National Commission for Certifying Agencies

NICU
Neonatal Intensive Care Unity

NP
Nurse Practitioner

OB
Obstetrics

OCN
Oncology Certified Nurse

OR
Operating Room

PA
Physician Assistant

PACU
Post-Anesthesia Care Unit

PCA
Personal Care Attendant

PICC
Peripherally Inserted Central Catheter

PICU
Pediatric Intensive Care Unit

PMHNP-BC
Psychiatric Mental Health Nurse Practitioner Board Certified

PNP
Pediatric Nurse Practitioner

PPE
Personal Protective Equipment

Preceptor
A person who guides, assists, and supports new or transferred nurses through orientation in a specific clinical area

PRN
pro re nata, Latin for "as needed"

PT
Physical Therapy

RN
Registered Nurse

RNC
Registered Nurse Certified

RYT
Registered Yoga Teacher

SDU
Step-Down Unit

SICU
Surgical Intensive Care Unit

SMART
Goals that are **S**pecific, **M**easurable, **A**chievable, **R**elevant, and **T**ime-bound

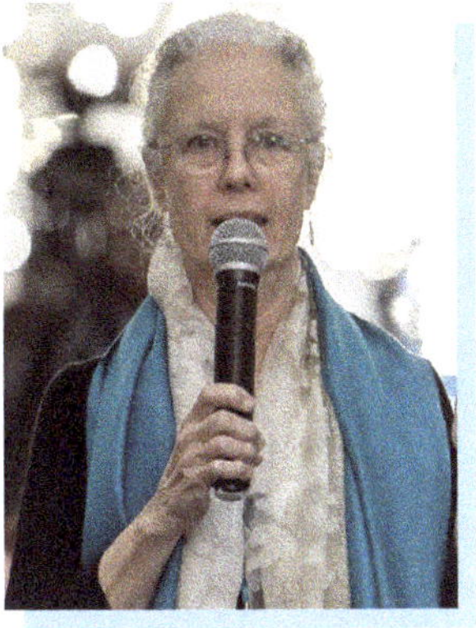

About the Author

Terry Maluk is a stress-management coach and author of multiple bestselling books that provide methods for learning to reduce stress and rediscover joy. A member of the American Holistic Nurses Association, Terry holds a Master of Science degree in Public Health, is an accredited, certified Emotional Freedom Techniques (EFT Tapping) practitioner, and a registered yoga teacher. Her extensive experience and her passion for helping others make her books excellent resources for anyone ready to start their journey toward a happier life.

FromStressedToCalm.com

Also by Terry Maluk

Rx for RNs: A Step-by-Step Guide to Manage Stress, Reduce Overwhelm, and Conquer Burnout

The Art of Managing Stress Series

Take One Breath: The Art of Managing Stress Through Mindful Breathing

In This Moment: The Art of Managing Stress Through Meditation

Emotional Freedom Techniques: The Art of Managing Stress Through EFT Tapping

CPSIA information can be obtained
at www.ICGtesting.com
Printed in the USA
BVHW092206230121
598512BV00003B/10

9 781732 772991